HIGHLY SENSITIVE EMPATH

HIGHLY SENSITIVE EMPATH

Copyright 2021 by Melissa Carroll - All rights reserved.

The content contained within this book may not be reproduced, duplicated or transmitted without direct written permission from the author or the publisher.

Under no circumstances will any blame or legal responsibility be held against the publisher, or author, for any damages, reparation, or monetary loss due to the information contained within this book. Either directly or indirectly.

Legal Notice:

This book is copyright protected. This book is only for personal use. You cannot amend, distribute, sell, use, quote or paraphrase any part, or the content within this book, without the consent of the author or publisher.

Disclaimer Notice:

Please note the information contained within this document is for educational and entertainment purposes only. All effort has been executed to present accurate, up to date, and reliable, complete information. No warranties of any kind are declared or implied. Readers acknowledge that the author is not engaging in the rendering of legal, financial, medical or professional advice. The content within this book has been derived from various sources. Please consult a licensed professional before attempting any techniques outlined in this book.

By reading this document, the reader agrees that under no circumstances is the author responsible for any losses, direct or indirect, which are incurred as a result of the use of information contained within this document, including, but not limited to, errors, omissions, or inaccuracies.

Table of Contents

PART ONE 8
INTRODUCTION 10
CHAPTER 1: THE JOURNEY TO BECOMING AN EMPATH 12
    THE EMPATHS AND SPIRITUALITY 13
    ARE YOU AN EMPATH? 14
CHAPTER 2: WHAT IS AN EMPATH? 16
CHAPTER 3: THE QUALITIES OF AN EMPATH 28
    POPULAR QUALITIES OF EMPATHS 29
    THE BRAIN AND THE EMPATH 33
    SYNAESTHESIA 37
CHAPTER 4: EMPATHS – THE GOOD, THE BAD AND THE UGLY ... 38
    BENEFITS OF BEING AN EMPATH 39
    CHALLENGES OF BEING AN EMPATH AND HOW TO OVERCOME
    THEM 43
    ANOTHER SIDE EFFECT THAT EMPATHS FACE IS A TRAIT THAT WAS
    MENTIONED EARLIER: LONELINESS 45
CHAPTER 5: TOOLS FOR TRANSFORMATION AND SPIRITUAL GROWTH 48
    WHAT IS SPIRITUALITY? 49
    DEVELOPING YOUR INTUITION 55
CHAPTER 6: EMPATHS AND ENERGY 60
    ROOT CHAKRA 61
    HOLY CHAKRA 62
    SOLAR PLEXUS CHAKRA 62
    THE HEART CHAKRA 62
    THE THROAT CHAKRA 63
    THE THIRD EYE CHAKRA 63
    THE CROWN CHAKRA 64
    HOW DO EMPATHS AFFECT ENERGY FLOWS? 64
    THE HEALING ENERGY FOR EMPATHS 66

CHAPTER 7: SELF-CARE FOR EMPATHS 70
TECHNIQUES FOR SELF-CARE 74

CHAPTER 8: HOW TO RE-CHANNEL YOUR EMPATH ENERGY 80
WHY AND HOW SHOULD WE LEARN TO REDIRECT ENERGY? 82
HOW TO HEAL AND PREVENT ENERGY BLOCKAGES 84

CHAPTER 9: THE GIFT OF HEALING AS AN EMPATH 90
THE COMMON TRAUMAS THAT EMPATHS EXPERIENCE 93
TECHNIQUES FOR EMPATHS HEALING 96

CHAPTER 10: HOW TO EMBRACE YOUR GIFT 100
HERE ARE SOME HELPFUL TIPS TO HELP YOU ACCEPT YOUR GIFT FULLY 101

CHAPTER 11: UNDERSTANDING THE IMPACT OF EMPATH ENERGY 104
MEDIUMISTIC SKILLS 105
PSYCHIC ABILITIES 109
ENERGY PROJECTION 109
HEALING 109

CHAPTER 12: EMPATHS AND SPIRITUAL HYPERSENSITIVITY 110
HOW TO COPE WITH SPIRITUAL HYPERSENSITIVITY 111
HOW TO USE ESSENTIAL OILS IN CALMING HYPERSENSITIVITY 118

CHAPTER 13: HOW EMPATHS DEAL WITH INSOMNIA, ADRENAL FATIGUE, AND EXHAUSTION 120
EFFECTS ON THE ADRENAL GLANDS 120
WHY YOU SHOULD CUT OUT REFINED SALT 123
WHY YOU SHOULD CUT OUT REFINED SUGAR 123

CHAPTER 14: HOW TO SHIELD YOURSELF FROM ENERGY VAMPIRES 128
DON'T GIVE TOO MUCH 128
REFRAIN FROM PLEASING PEOPLE 129
BE WARY OF THE GREEDY PEOPLE 129
BE MINDFUL OF NEEDY PEOPLE 129
LOOK OUT FOR DRAMA QUEENS 129
CLARITY 130
HERB SMUDGING 130
CRYSTALS AND GEMSTONES OR GEM ELIXIRS 130
ORGONE 130

- THE CANDLES 131
- INCENSE AND RESINS 131
- FOR BATHS 131
- PROTECTION CHANTS AND PRAYERS 131

CHAPTER 15: EMPATHS AND HOW THEY FUNCTION AT WORK. 132

- ASK FOR A TOUR OF THE WORKPLACE BEFORE TAKING UP A JOB132
- USING YOUR GIFT AS A SELLING POINT 133
- WORKING ALONE VERSUS WORKING WITH OTHERS 133
- IF YOU'RE IN AN ENVIRONMENT THAT DRAINS ENERGY, ASK FOR REASONABLE ADJUSTMENTS 134
- LOOK OUT FOR ENERGY VAMPIRE 135
- CREATE BOUNDARIES BETWEEN YOUR WORKPLACE AND YOUR HOME 136
- FOCUS ON HOW YOUR WORK WILL BENEFITS OTHERS 137

CHAPTER 16: HOW TO NORMALIZE AND MAINTAIN YOUR EMPATH GIFT 138

- PRESERVE YOUR GIFT 139
- CHECK-IN REGULARLY 139
- DAILY MEDITATION 140
- DEEP BREATHING 140
- DELIBERATE GROUNDING 141

CHAPTER 17: NURTURE YOUR OWN ENERGY 142

- ALIGNING WITH THE FORCE OF GRACE 143
- ESTABLISH A CHECKLIST FOR INTIMACY 146
- PRACTICE RADICAL SELF-LOVE 148
- RECOGNIZE INTENSE, NEUTRAL OR MILD ENERGY 149
- GOSSIP DETOX 150
- RELEASE SOMEONE WITH LOVE 151
- CONFRONT OTHERS WHILE YOU DEFEND YOURSELF 153

CHAPTER 18: HOW TO SUPPORT A YOUNG EMPATH 156

- HOW TO SPOT A YOUNG EMPATH 156
- REVEAL THE REAL MOTIVES BEHIND TEMPER TANTRUMS 157
- BUILD A FRIENDLY ENVIRONMENT 158
- HELP THEM TO PLAN FOR THE HARSHER REALITIES OF LIFE 159
- GIVING THEM REALISTIC APPROACHES THAT THEY CAN USE 160
- TEENAGER EMPATHS 161

CHAPTER 19: KEEPING YOUR EMPATH SPACE CLEAN AND UNCLUTTERED 164
- BE INTENTIONAL ABOUT YOUR DECORATIONS 165
- CREATING COMFORTABLE ENERGY 166
- CLEAR THE ENERGY OF YOUR SPACE 167

CONCLUSION PART ONE 170

PART TWO 174

INTRODUCTION 176

CHAPTER 20: WHAT IS PSYCHIC POWER AND HOW CAN YOU DISCOVER YOUR INTUITIVE TYPE? 178
- THE FOUR PSYCHIC INTUITION STYLES 183

CHAPTER 21: THE WORLD OF PROFESSIONAL PSYCHICS 192
- STEREOTYPES 194
- 1-800 HOTLINES 194
- HOW TO SPOT SCAM ARTISTS 196
- IDENTIFYING WHO IS WHO 198
- MISCONCEPTIONS ABOUT PSYCHICS AND THEIR ABILITIES ... 198
- MISCONCEPTIONS 200

CHAPTER 22: HOW TO IMPROVE YOUR MENTAL HEALTH 208

CHAPTER 23: PSYCHIC PROTECTION 222

CHAPTER 24: CLAIRVOYANT HEALING 234

CHAPTER 25: PSYCHIC EMPATH AND TELEPATHY 240

CHAPTER 26: THE ART OF GUIDED MEDITATION 246

CHAPTER 27: COMMUNICATING WITH SPIRIT GUIDES 252

CHAPTER 28: THE BIGGEST PROS AND CONS OF BEING A PSYCHIC EMPATH 256
- WHAT IS AN EMPATH? 256
- THE PROS AND CONS 257
- THE PLEASURES AND PITFALLS OF BECOMING AN EMPATH ... 259
- SEVEN IMPORTANT PRACTICES FOR EMPATHS 261

CHAPTER 29: ALL YOU NEED TO KNOW ABOUT ENERGY VAMPIRES 264
- WHAT IS AN ENERGY VAMPIRE? 264
- SIGNS OF BAD ENERGY IN YOUR LIFE AND HOW TO CLEAR IT OUT 270

SIGNS OF NEGATIVE ENERGY IN YOUR LIFE 271
  HOW TO GET RID OF NEGATIVE ENERGY 272
  HOW TO DETOX YOUR HOME OF BAD ENERGY 274

CHAPTER 30: THE ROLE OF MEDIUMSHIP AND PSYCHIC EMPATH 276

CHAPTER 31: DREAM INTERPRETATION FOR A PSYCHIC EMPATH 280

CHAPTER 32: PSYCHIC DEVELOPMENT EXERCISES FOR EMPATHS 294

  GATHERING LIKE-MINDED PEOPLE..294
  TURNING YOUR ABILITIES ON AND OFF..295
  THE EXERCISES..297

CHAPTER 33: HOW TO CONTINUE WITH YOUR PSYCHIC EMPATH DEVELOPMENT 310

  READING AND MEDITATION 311

CHAPTER 34: SOME FINAL TIPS 322

  PROVING YOURSELF..322
  WE'RE NOT FORTUNE COOKIES 323
  AVOIDING DEPENDENCY..326
  FRIENDS AND ACQUANTANCES 327
  LET YOUR LIGHT SHINE...328

CONCLUSION PART TWO 330

Part One

INTRODUCTION

Greetings my dear readers! Congratulations on taking the first step toward excellence as you continue to recognize and use your gift for the common good! If you're reading this, I can only presume you're new and have just become aware of your gift as an empath. You are probably both scared and excited; scared because you don't fully get it and excited because you're about to move into a new world of possibilities you didn't have any idea about.

Empaths who cannot control their gift learn that it is a horrible source of tension, anxiety, and pain. Feeling the feelings of other people as though they were your own might feel like you're on a constant roller coaster of emotions. The purpose of this book is to take you to a place of rest with regard to the gift you have been blessed with. You're going to discover just what your talent is, and why you're so fortunate.

I want you to realize that you bear tremendous strength, and the dynamism of it is the reason why it affects you in such a profound way. There are many advantages and blessings associated with being an empath, and doors of opportunity will begin to open for you as you learn to step in and accept your gift.

Take your time before moving on to the next, to fully understand and absorb each chapter. Prepare your mind for the keys you'll find in this book to open the wealth of promise that's within you. I highly encourage you to join our tight-knit group on Facebook to maximize the value that you gain from this book. To continue your development, you will be able to connect and share with other like-minded empaths here. It is not advisable to take this path alone and this could be an exceptional support network for you.

CHAPTER 1:

THE JOURNEY TO BECOMING AN EMPATH

Have you ever felt like a fault was being understood? Are you always made to weep by the sight of other people weeping, regardless of what it is about? Do you enjoy spending time with other people after social experiences but find yourself feeling overwhelmed or drained? Should you think of yourself as an introvert? If you are connected to this, then you could be what is known as an empath. In this book, we'll discuss what empath means, how this is a gift, and how you can grow the ability further.

If you are reading this book, you would probably have been either classified as an empath or think that you might be a highly sensitive person. If you are unfamiliar with any of these words, you may just want to be more in tune with yourself, your surroundings, and how you relate to others. Recently, the word "empath" has become important to mainstream culture, as more individuals become conscious of how they could contribute to this form of personality. In an era of social media, it is impossible not to get obsessed by other people's thoughts and emotions. You can find yourself a little frustrated if you constantly check your Twitter to see news updates about all the tragedies going on in the world. This is understandable because constant stimulation can be exhausting and overwhelming, particularly emotionally charged stimulation.

It is incredibly natural for empaths to feel this, as they continually take in the emotions of other people, and as we adapt to a stimulating world of emotions being shared online and on social media, more and more people identify as empaths. It can seem difficult to avoid this, simply because each time we open our phones or turn the news on we are surrounded by emotions being thrown at us. Identifying as an empath isn't inherently a bad thing, though.

It can sometimes be called a gift, in reality. You will cultivate this talent and succeed socially as an empath with the right understanding and self-care tools. An empath is commonly described as a person who is able to internalize other people's feelings around them. Obviously, the term relates to the principle of an empath, which is defined as the capacity to understand and even feel the emotions of other people. Although humans are usually capable of experiencing empathy, including feeling sorry for a friend when they lose a loved one, being an empath is less normal. Empaths sense this feeling to the point that they are unable to control it and can perceive other people's emotions to almost the same degree.

Although the two words are associated, it is important to distinguish that a person does not become empathic merely by experiencing empath. Empaths identify as individuals who experience a great deal of empath all the time, even to the point that they feel exhausted or frustrated. They are also over-stimulated and unable to suppress such stimuli in the way that others would. There are numerous psychological characteristics that lead to empath, which we will discuss in later chapters. Simply put, however, because of their hypersensitive nerves, empaths store emotions, and energy differently.

THE EMPATHS AND SPIRITUALITY

Being an empath is also related to various aspects of spirituality as well. Being an empath is seen as a sort of superpower, as established in the science fiction universe. Many people agree that empaths are far more in touch with other people's thoughts and energies and are able to internalize them, which can combine well with energy healing or other activities that involve a deep understanding of the emotions of another person. Some also claim it can be a sign of having psychic skills to be an empath. Empaths have an exceptionally powerful understanding of the energies of other people, making them good spiritual and clairvoyant healers.

According to psychiatrist Judith Orloff, who has carried out extensive studies on the psychiatry behind the empath and describes herself as an empath, empath is also very sensitive to the energy that flows in and out of humans. High levels of intuition can also be encountered by empaths, but these gifts are not always promoted and can be suppressed in childhood and early adulthood (Mason, 2005). We will discuss in later chapters how to cultivate innate abilities that have been hidden, and how to become more conscious of the way our brains can pick up on the energies of other people. In addition, even non-empaths can train themselves to become more empathetic and receptive to the emotions and energies of other people, which may encourage us to learn some of those skills even if they do not come as naturally.

ARE YOU AN EMPATH?

You have probably chosen this book, as described earlier because you think you might be an empath. You may also be interested in the energies behind empath and want to learn more about how intuition gifts can be created. We will look into what makes a person an empath in the next few chapters, how to grow and use your empath while preventing burnout, and how the empath of a person can interact with different spiritual practices.

You may consider yourself a Highly Sensitive Person (HSP) even if you don't completely classify yourself as an empath. HSPs also show many of the same characteristics since empaths, as in all groups of people, certain functions of the brain function the same way. This book will also allow you to improve your empath, if this is the case for you, while still being able to escape the burnout that can come with being highly sensitive.

If you're always uncertain as to whether you're an empath, that's all right. In these next few pages, we'll further discuss what becoming an empath entails and how it affects your life. And if you're not completely sure you're an empath, that's good too! Empath is an emotion that can be further created, and you can also use it as an instrument to progress in your own forms of spirituality.

CHAPTER 2:

WHAT IS AN EMPATH?

An empath is a person with an accessible spirit; in the unseen and the seen world, they unconsciously feel things to the point that they may become a burden. They absorb the energy that affects them and have a natural ability to respond to other people's feelings. They're affected by the moods, emotions, expectations, and wishes of other people. Having an empath isn't limited to high sensitivity and emotions; they know others' motives and motivations intuitively. Empath is not something that is taught; either you are born that way or you are not. As an empath, you are continually in contact with other people's emotions and thoughts, ensuring you are continually bearing the weight of those around you.

The physical manifestations of the feelings they are burdened with, such as regular aches and pains and persistent tiredness, are vulnerable to multiple empaths. I am sure you heard the saying, "You look like you're holding on your shoulders the weight of the world!" This is what the empath is doing! They bear everybody's powers, emotions, and karma that they come into contact with. Empaths are highly humble; they shy away from compliments and tend to thank someone else rather than accept them. They express themselves with great enthusiasm and communicate with great frankness, which can often trigger the offense. They're not the kind of individuals who mask their feelings; they're going to open up to everyone who wants to listen.

They can also be the complete opposite on the other side of this; they can be very anti-social and would happily block those that they believe are hindering them in any way from their lives. They do not know why they do this; this is also their way of blocking out the emotions and energies they continually have to contend with from others to the empath who may not understand who they are.

Although empaths are sensitive to other people's feelings, they don't spend much time listening to their own hearts. This can lead them before their own to care for the needs of others. Usually, an empath is non-aggressive, non-violent, and is fast to become the peacemaker between individuals. When they are in an atmosphere of disharmony, an empath feels incredibly uncomfortable; they avoid conflict or make adjustments quickly if a situation gets out of control. They hate themselves for it and will make a fast apology if they lose control and say something that would cause offense.

Empaths appear to pick up others' emotions and then project them back to the person without understanding what they're doing. When an empath is in the early stages of recognizing their gift, it's recommended that they talk things out to release the build-up of emotions. If not, they prefer to bottle things up and build walls of skyscrapers around themselves, refusing to let others in. The inability to communicate their feelings is often the product of a traumatic incident, a childhood in which emotions were not expressed at home, or parents who instructed them to see and not hear them.

Emotional detachment can have a detrimental impact on our health; the more control they have over us, the longer we keep our emotions inside without release. There will finally be a release as feelings build-up, and that release is a positive thing. Man is programmed to express himself when he feels a burden; that is how healing occurs. When you chat things out, there's an emotional relief; you don't bear the weight alone anymore. There is a chance of mental and emotional instability as well as negative feelings manifesting in the form of an illness if this does not take place.

Empaths are sensitive to film, television, photographs, and news shows showing scenes of violence or physical or emotional pain and distress, whether adult, child, or animal. This can bring them down to tears and cause them to get physically sick. For those who do not have the same degree of humanity as they do, they are unable to explain the pain they experience and see and have little tolerance.

Empaths work in professions that encourage them, whether it's with animals, nature, or people, to assist others. They are passionate about their jobs and their contribution to others. Empaths are also found in volunteer roles that dedicate their time to helping others without pay or recognition. Empaths are excellent storytellers because of their ceaseless imagination; they are always learning and asking questions. They are also very gentle and romantic; they are sentimental about family history and will keep old memories, jewelry, or other valuables passed down from generations. Sometimes, they are the ones who sit and listen to stories shared by grandparents and great grandparents and have a wealth of knowledge about their family's past.

They listen to a range of music styles to accommodate the array of moods they're feeling. People are often curious about their musical taste, especially the degree of diversity. They listen to classical music for one minute and in the next hardcore rap! The lyrics to a song can have a powerful impact on an empath, especially if it relates to something they have recently encountered. To prevent sending their feelings into a spin, it is recommended that empaths listen to music without lyrics.

Empaths use their body language as a mean of expression; through dance, body gestures, and acting, they can communicate themselves as easily as they can through words. Empaths, as they dance, are able to show high volumes of energy; they get lost in the music and enter a trance-like state as their spirits sync with the beat and the lyrics. They characterize the feeling as being totally lost in the moment; they are no longer conscious of others' presence.

Empaths have spirits that are really beautiful, so people are naturally attracted to them without knowing why. They can notice that total strangers feel comfortable sharing the most personal subjects and interactions with them. Another explanation why an empath is so magnetic is because it's really good listeners; it's bubbly, outgoing, enthusiastic, and people want to be there. They are the life and soul of any group, and because they feed off their energy, individuals like to have them around. The reverse is also valid because of the intense nature of their character; their moods will shift in an instant, and people will scatter like cockroaches to get away from them. The responsibility of bearing too many emotions can be daunting if an empath cannot appreciate their talent. They do not realize why they feel the feelings of someone else; it is frustrating for them. They are good for one moment and the next, they experience a flood of depression, which causes them to act out.

It's not a smart idea to sacrifice empath in one of their mood swings in the heights. Whoever is around at this time should give them a shoulder to sob, be sympathetic, and be an ear to listen. Sometimes, this return of emphatic emotional treatment will lead to an imminent recovery. Empaths are often mistaken, and it is a vital part of their journey that they do, as well as those around them, do not only understand themselves.

Empaths are also learners and solvers of problems; they love to research a number of different materials. They assume that there are problems and solutions together, and that a solution is always at hand. Sometimes they will look until they find the solution to a dilemma that can be of great help to those around them, whether at work or at home. An empath is also capable of tapping into universe information and seeking advice to solve the dilemma they've put their minds to.

Empaths are dreamers; the dreams are vivid and informative. They assume that their dreams are connected to their actual life and that something that is happening in their lives or the lives of someone they know is being warned about. They have spent their time and commitment from a young age in unlocking the secrets of their dreams.

Empaths thrive off mental engagement; they have no desire for the worldly, and find it hard to concentrate on things that do not inspire them. They will also resort to daydreaming and settle into a disconnected state of mind when they find themselves becoming bored. While their physical body is in the same place, they have another dimension to their mind.

If they are as articulate and emotional as they are, an instructor will only maintain the attention of an empathic student; if not, they will turn off easily. If their audience doesn't fully captivate the empaths, they lack interest. Because of their inherent capacity to become so submerged by the emotions of others, they produce the best actors that when they perform a part, they do so with all the emotions of the character they play.

They are vulnerable to synchronicities and déjà vu being witnessed. What starts out as a series of continuous coincidences leads to an interpretation of who empath is to see into the future. When this recognition becomes a reality, they begin to communicate with the power of their gift, a feeling of euphoria sets in.

Many empaths have a strong connection to the paranormal; throughout their lives, they may have a variety of near-death and out-of-body encounters. Traveling to another world of the spirit realm is a natural occurrence in the life of an empath. They are free spirits and what they live for is not the mundane routine of life. When they get caught in this loop, the sense of life is lost, and they are forced to pause, re-examine their lives, and return to self-discovery on their journey. Their paranormal encounters contribute to isolation; this is not the rule for the average person, and so empaths tend to inhibit their abilities in fear of being unfairly branded. However, they can resolve this, and it generally occurs when they are surrounded by other empaths.

There are a number of empaths, each using a different psychic emphatic characteristic. They are exactly as follows:

1. **Geomancy**: Geomancers have the power to sense the energy of the earth; they can feel the energy when they are on certain land and in some locations. They get headaches when a natural disaster is about to take place, regardless of where it is happening.

2. **Telepathy:** They have the power to hear others' minds.

3. **Psychometry:** They may get energy from perceptions, locations, photos, or artifacts.

4. **Physical healing:** The capacity to experience in their own body the physical effects of others, which they can then use to facilitate healing.

5. **Animal communication:** The capacity to sense, hear, and interact with animals.

6. **Emotional healing:** The capacity to sense others' feelings.

7. **Nature:** Capacity to interact with plants and nature.

8. **Mediumship**: The ability to sense the force of spirits and their presence.

9. **Awareness or claircognizance**: The ability to realize what must be done in any given situation; in the middle of a crisis, this is frequently combined with a sense of calm and peace.

10. **Precognition:** The ability to feel that a significant event is about to happen. There is also a sense of gloom or fear that is mysterious.

If you are unsure as to whether or not you have an empathic gift, here are 25 typical features of empath:

1. They are searching for the survivor, the underdog; those who are going through mental pain and misery are attracting the empath's attention.

2. The empath is extremely imaginative with a vibrant imagination; the ability to sing, dance, draw, act, or compose is typically multitalented. An untidy world full of confusion and mess blocks the flow of empathic energy; they're really minimalistic and clean.

3. They have a disregard for narcissism. Although empaths are very tolerant, compassionate, and sweet, they don't like being around greedy characters who exist for themselves and have little respect for others' feelings and emotions.

4. In food, they sense energy. Empaths are also vegetarian since the pain endured by the animal when being slaughtered can be felt.

5. They don't want to buy second-hand items, because they feel that their energy is carried by something already owned by another. They choose to buy a brand new house or a brand new car when the empath is financially secure, so they don't get into someone else's energy.

6. They spend daydreaming time. An empath with their own imagination can get lost; they can gladly stare for hours with oblivion. They get bored and distracted when an empath isn't stimulated. Whether at home, at work, or at school, they have

to be involved in what they're doing, or they're going to wander.

7. They are pursuers of information. Empaths still learn something new; if they have unanswered questions, they find it challenging, and they will go beyond and beyond the call of duty to find the answer. They will look for confirmation if they sense a nudge in their spirit that they have an answer. The downside to this is that they hold so much information, which can be exhausting. They have a strong desire to discover, as we discover it, more about the universe.

8. They can't indulge in something they're not loving. When they participate in things that they don't like, they feel as though they are not honest about themselves. Many empaths are classified as lazy because they refuse to take part in something in which they do not agree, and most things tend to be that.

9. The need for loneliness. They have to get time alone, which is true also with children with empath.

10. They have a passion for nature and animals. Empaths love life and being at one with nature outdoors. Usually, they have pets inside the property. They think plants and animals have thoughts and feelings.

11. They are very much in contact with the spiritual world, and things are common for them, such as seeing ghosts and spirits. They also tend to have access to data that scientists would spend years attempting to accomplish. Empaths, for instance, understood the world was round while everyone else thought it was flat.

12. They are still tired; they feel continually exhausted and tired, because they are so vulnerable to the energy of others. This

exhaustion is so severe that they can't even be healed by sleep. Empaths are sometimes diagnosed with Myalgic Encephalomyelitis (ME). They have back issues and stomach disorders. The middle of the abdomen is where the chakra of the solar plexus is positioned. In this area, empaths feel the feelings of others, which weakens them and may contribute to irritable bowel syndrome, stomach ulcers, and lower back problems. Usually, the empath who does not appreciate their gift may suffer from such physical issues. They catch diseases quickly; the physical symptoms of those around them grow an empath. They also catch the body and joints from the flu, eye infections, and aches and pains. Often they feel compassion pains when they're close to others.

13. An empath is a sounding board. All goes empathically to unload their issues, sometimes winding up as their own. They sense the feelings of others and take them on. They can sense the emotions of those near, far, or both. The more practiced an empath understands that someone feels poorly about them.

14. They can pinpoint lies. The empath is conscious when someone doesn't tell the truth, and when someone thinks or feels one way but tells something else they know. To know that they are lying, they don't need to listen to the sound of someone's voice or examine their facial expressions; they have the ability to instinctively know whether or not they are lying.

15. They find it hard to witness some form of aggression. Neither do they read about it in newspapers and magazines; as a result, empaths find it hard to watch television or to read newspapers and magazines.

16. Sometimes they get confused in public areas. It is difficult for the empath to be in areas like stores, stadiums, and shopping centers where there are a lot of people because of the amount

of energy emitted from the crowds. Their setting is structured and planned to function around their sensitivities. To avoid unpredictable, uncomfortable conditions that are too challenging, their timetable and duties are structured.

17. They have access to cutting-edge information. Empaths are tailored to knowledge; they know stuff without saying it. This is not intuition or feeling in the gut, their awareness comes from a greater source of influence. The greater this gift becomes, the more they are tuned into their gift.

18. They're able to affect people's moods. They are very charismatic, and their enthusiasm attracts individuals. They start talking and behaving much like them when they spend too much time with people.

19. They love being around the water; they love the vitality of the oceans, the rivers, the seas.

20. They have always been told they are too fragile and too emotional. Their ability to pick up on emotions and signs isn't natural for anyone else, but it's theirs.

21. They have poor pain tolerance; when they have to deal with even the slightest of injuries, they find it hard to get injections and feel sick. They might also be advised by doctors that they complain too much.

22. They are very observant in reading facial expressions and body language, and are exceptionally fine.

23. They are drawn to healing professions; nurses, physicians, or veterinarians are also empaths. Empaths are attracted to become counselors, social workers, communicators of animals, teachers, and carers.

24. Empaths are drawn to complementary and healing arts, such as organic foods, hypnotherapy, psychotherapy, holistic practices, energy and Reiki, and psychic reading. They have a philosophical interest, such as prayer, meditation, yoga, and positive affirmations.

25. They are non-conformists who want to live beyond the constraints of the work standard of society—a family and kids. They love traveling, freedom, and adventure. Empaths are free spirits; they do not like stagnation. Laws, routine, or power, they don't like. An empath likes having the right to do whatever they want to do when they want to. They feel constrained and imprisoned if they are unable to do so.

CHAPTER 3:

THE QUALITIES OF AN EMPATH

One of the key attributes of an empath, in its conventional context, is sensitivity. Empaths have neural functions that are extremely sensitive, allowing them to feel high levels of stimulation. While most individuals are able to filter out stimuli and choose what they want to concentrate on instead, empaths are unable to do so.

They feel everything basically, picking up on all the energies around them. Because of this, empaths can very easily become over-stimulated and confused. This may also render them particularly vulnerable to emotional infection, which can frequently occur in large groups. The phenomenon can also be observed by non-empaths. Have you ever noticed how you can often become irritable or nervous when someone is especially on-edge around you? But this is an even more serious occurrence for empaths and something that is really hard to filter out. That is yet another example of why empath typically needs to spend time alone to recharge and ground itself. Many features of becoming an empath are items that occur in non-empaths, but in a much higher form, as we will discuss in this chapter.

Empaths and Higly Sensitive People, in short, vary from individuals who do not associate with these groups because of the way their brains function. Empaths and HSPs have hyper-sensitive neurons which cause them to internalize other people's pain and emotions, often to the same extent. However, they are not generally aware of the phenomenon occurring in their brain which causes them to do so. In addition, while empaths share all the qualities of HSPs, by being able to pick up on the subtle energies of people and internalize them, they take these qualities further. Because of this significant difference, we will concentrate not only on the daily aspects of becoming an empath, but also on the unique metaphysical processes that empaths are also able to perform. Later in this chapter, we'll discuss the functions in our brains that make us feel empathic. Let's first analyze, however, how these roles express themselves in our actions and feelings so that we can discuss the popular characteristics of empaths.

Since the notion of becoming an empath is a relatively recent concept, as it relates to other facets of the personality of an individual, we should address empath. The Big Five scale is one scale widely used to measure personality. The attributes measured on this scale are openness, conscientiousness, extraversion, neuroticism, and agreeability. As they relate to an empath and the notion of empath, these characteristics are often brought up, although the existence of empath in an individual can differ. It is also noticed, however, that individuals who classify as empaths often have high levels of conscientiousness, and those with disabilities marked by low levels of empath typically have lower levels of conscientiousness. As we examine what it means to be an empath, we'll address the various ways a person's personality is made up of common traits.

POPULAR QUALITIES OF EMPATHS

Orloff, who has done extensive empathic research, has produced a shortlist of several common empathic characteristics to help people decide whether they identify as empathic. We will explore in-depth some of these traits to help you decide whether you are an empath, or if you have some of the traits of an empath that you could create. It is possible to see all of these characteristics together, since many empaths can perceive one attribute as a result of another. Some traits, however, don't evolve immediately. While empaths are very intuitive and have basic instincts to use their emotions, due to circumstances, many empathic qualities develop. Although researchers once assumed that empath is an intrinsic capacity that can not be taught, it is now thought that empathic abilities can be produced and, depending on circumstances, can alter. In this regard, the way we interpret and communicate our emotions, as well as the emotions of others, will influence our environments and the people we associate ourselves with.

Empaths share several characteristics with highly sensitive individuals, as described earlier. Hence one aspect of an empath is highly sensitive. Have you ever been told you're "too sensitive? Can you feel that things that happen to other people and are told that you "care too much" have a very personal effect on yourself? You could be an empath then. Empaths internalize their thoughts as much as those of other persons, experiencing them deeply. If you think that you are particularly sensitive to stimuli, then you are definitely an empath. This can be either emotional stimulus or even simply heightened senses being heard.

Empaths are often vulnerable, particularly in large crowds and social settings, to sensory overload. Empaths are often known to hate big crowds and small talk, because of the overwhelming sensation that large stimuli can create. Since an empath takes too much in and has a hard time managing what stimuli their brains do and don't react to, circumstances where there's a lot going on, like large meetings or huge crowds, can be really stressful and exhausting. Empaths are often also nervous and/or introverted, mainly because it can be difficult for them to be around people. In order to recharge, it is common for empaths to need time alone. It can also go hand in hand with social anxiety, as because of the constant activity going on in their minds, empaths can become nervous around other individuals.

Another common feature of an empath is to take on or internalize the feelings of other people. Although most people can, to a certain degree, experience empath, empaths can fully absorb the feelings of another person and feel the emotions as though they are their own. It's normal for someone, for instance, to understand and feel sad about a friend who just broke up with their significant other. An empath, however, will take this grief a step further and genuinely feel the suffering of their friend as though it were their own. If you often feel the suffering of others around you as if it were your own, then you are possibly an empath.

This can also go for other emotions, but an empath can also have difficulty identifying where the feelings of another person end and theirs begin. Have you ever spent time, for example, with someone who wouldn't stop moaning about something going wrong with their lives, and then you came home in a bad mood? This is a trait of empath, as they appear to internalize other people's feelings around them. It also means they are able to pick up and process other people's energy, which can also mean that after spending time with unpleasant people, they find themselves in a bad mood.

As mentioned earlier, the most frequently defined as introverts are empaths. An introvert is someone who gets their energy from spending time alone, while extroverts get energy from spending time with others. Empaths also become exhausted and, after social activities, need to rest and so enjoy spending time alone. Empaths in large groups often run out of steam, and often prefer spending time with one or a few individuals instead of spending time in large groups. Empaths often avoid large groups of individuals, and sometimes feel very frustrated, thereby making them vulnerable to social anxiety. This may sound like a paradox, as an empath is very people-oriented and is a natural caretaker and help. Nevertheless, they are introverts in the sense that when they are around people too often, they believe their vitality is drained. This is because they consume the energy of other people, but still bring a great deal of their own energy into others, causing them to feel exhausted and drained.

In addition, feeling like you are an outsider or may not fit in with other individuals is another quality of being an empath. While empaths are extremely sensitive and emotionally in line with the feelings of other people, this may end up contributing to feelings of isolation. Many who consider as powerful empaths will find that other individuals do not feel as strongly as they do, leading them not to have anything in common. That can contribute to pushing away others and feelings of loneliness. Empaths may also have difficulty maintaining romantic or close relationships. This may be because it may become difficult to discern the distinction between their own emotions and the emotions of the other person that they have internalized as they get close to others.

Moreover, especially if the other person is extremely hostile, it can place a toll on the personal feelings and vibrational field of empath. This can allow negative energy to become internalized by empath. Because of this, empaths may prefer to avoid being intimate and/or close to others. They then sometimes end up pushing away and/or isolating other individuals, which can lead to isolation or the feeling of becoming an outsider. Empaths must first prioritize their interactions with themselves before pouring all their resources into other individuals. Although this may feel like you're isolating yourself at first, it will, in fact, be helpful in the long run as focusing on establishing a positive relationship with yourself is a good basis for developing strong and healthy relationships with others. By concentrating on your internal energies, you will find that you will be far more in charge of the external energy that you are transmitting and even internalizing, which in turn will have beneficial effects on several different areas of your life.

Although all of these appear to be typical side effects of empath, an empath often appears to have hyperactive senses, making them vulnerable to sensory overload. In addition to other characteristics of being extremely sensitive, if you find yourself frustrated by sounds or smells, you may describe yourself as an empath. Empaths, in addition, also gravitate to nature. Nature can be energizing to empaths, equivalent to recharging in solitude. Interestingly enough, an empath is also drawn into the water as well. Water appears to energize them, and it can help to restore the empath by being near a large body of water. You may identify as an empath if you recognize any or several of these common signs in yourself, particularly in conjunction with each other. Let's now explore how certain tendencies and qualities can be generated by the functions of an empathic brain.

THE BRAIN AND THE EMPATH

Human beings have evolved brains through evolution that are highly capable of picking up on others' feelings, including subtle ones. In reality, we have become so capable of this that some of us can not only feel the emotions and energies of others but internalize them as if they are ours. Many scientists suggest that in order to create and care for their children, humans evolved the capacity to empathize. Researchers have also found evidence of this quality in other mammals that, relative to non-mammals, produce a smaller number of offspring.

Although we may be genetically predisposed to experience some kind of empath, other factors, like how we are raised and the environment we live in, may influence how this quality develops further. Although some researchers claim that the amount of empath we display as children is the same amount we will have for the remainder of our lives, others claim that empath can be easily created and increased. Another common speculation is that humans have developed empath for mutualism purposes which helps the entire species to survive and continue to reproduce.

Researchers have found that people, even unintentionally, appear to mimic each other's behavior. This can translate into feelings and emotions, as a person can see someone else experiencing sorrow and then experience it on their own. We normally, however, feel the feelings of others to a lesser degree in order not to let it overwhelm us. For example, if you were to find out that your friend is feeling grief over a bad break-up, you would probably be sad for them too, but you wouldn't spend as much time grieving their relationship end as they would. This is because our brains are wired in a way that decreases the degree to which we feel the same emotions to respond to these stimuli. In the end, this helps us to be more supportive to the person suffering from pain. But the response is different for empaths. Empaths are much more responsive to these sensations, allowing them to experience the discomfort to a greater extent than most individuals. This can result in them feeling others' suffering at a level almost equal to how it is felt by the person experiencing the hardship.

Many scientists agree that the empath has multiple components to it. One aspect is a reaction to the feelings and/or actions of another person, always experiencing what they feel. The next aspect is the ability to cognitively follow the perspective of the other person while addressing a topic. Finally, psychologists conclude that the behavior of controlling one's own thoughts on the matter requires empath. We can see how the minds of empaths are basically working overtime to absorb the thoughts of those around them by studying the various neural mechanisms that go into experiencing empath.

Although all these various components that go into the empath are encountered by most empathic individuals, empaths experience them in a heightened way, hence the reason that they function overtime. Their brains are fundamentally wired differently in order not only to control their own feelings about the emotions of the other person they are feeling but also to internalize the emotions as their own. This is why it is so important for empaths to start recognizing the energies and feelings that they first internalize before acting on them. This will affect the way they will then control their own thoughts and feelings as a result of the energy they gather from other people.

The definition of self-awareness is another neural component of empath that varies between empaths and non-empaths. This is an essential component of empath because it prevents emotional contagion or the inability to separate the emotions of another person from one's own. This is the field where people struggle with empath. Clearly, an empath is very good at understanding and acting on the feelings of other people, but it is very vulnerable to emotional contagion. In addition, many of the neural mechanisms that decide how we experience empath are related to our own viewpoint, which is analogous to self-awareness in that it is an appreciation of our different points of view. This is also another definition that differs in terms of empath. While several researchers suggest that we are more inclined to empathize with those we connect to or share with us a mutual purpose, empaths, regardless of their connection, may empathize with everyone. The definition of empath has two extremes. Someone who feels as much empath as possible is called an empath, as we have already developed.

There are, however, some personality disorders in which humans have little or no empath for others. Narcissists and psychopaths include individuals who show very little empath for others. Looking at the biological functions behind empath, the distinction between an empath and a psychopath or a narcissist is the way our mirror neurons operate. The brain's response to witnessing feelings and responses in other individuals is mediated by mirror neurons.

The hypothesis that these neurons can potentially replicate what someone is feeling in our own minds has been created by scientists so that we can empathize directly with them. According to this theory, our minds are simply trying to mimic what they are going through while we empathize with others so that we can perceive and/or feel the same thing in essence. This relates to the notion of self-awareness again. There is something of an overlap in our brains between our self-centered processes and processes centered on others. This helps one to empathize with others through the internalization of their feelings to understand them.

Empaths possibly have a greater connection between self-focused and other-focused systems, frequently internalizing the thoughts of others as their own. Using the principle of simulation, we will also begin to understand why empaths are so vulnerable to their energy being overwhelmed or drained. Burnout may seem unavoidable when one is continually simulating another person's thoughts and emotions in their own brain.

Another element of empath to remember is that many experts in psychology agree that there are two forms of empath encountered by humans: physical, and cognitive. In order to feel sympathy for them, relational empath defines the ways in which we can internalize another person's feelings. This is at the core of altruism, generally described as selfless in the pursuit of other people's welfare. When we feel sad because our friends are sad, our emotional empath is at play. Of course, this is a common feature of empath, since they are very sensitive to feelings and can feel them profoundly, even though they are not their own.

The second form of empath, cognitive empath, refers to how we can precisely perceive and establish a correct understanding of the emotions of another person. This will manifest, using the same example, in how we might be able to understand that our friend is sad, why they are sad, and how they are sad instead of angry. We describe the relationship between one's actions and emotions through the cognitive processes. For example, cognitive empath will be at play when we understand that our friend recently distanced himself from us and was not present at social events (their behavior) because they're depressed about a recent break-up they've undergone (their emotions). Empaths are normally proficient in both moral and cognitive compassion. They are usually quite in line with human behavior, because they can use observations to understand human emotion, even though it has not been expressly shown. They can also internalize the feelings of another person, and mimic what they feel, demonstrating that they have a high degree of emotional empath.

Although many empaths may refer to the internalization of the emotions of others as their own, recent psychological research has found that only 1-2 % of the population consists of what are called "super empaths." Super empaths can not only simulate other people's feelings, but also experience their actual feelings literally. This kind of empathic trait is often referred to as mirror-touch synesthesia ("Super Empaths"), according to a 2018 research presentation at the ERSC's Festival of Social Sciences.

SYNAESTHESIA

Synaesthesia is characterized as a disorder in which it becomes difficult to differentiate two or more senses. You may have encountered anyone, for instance, who claims that some sounds have a color about them. This is an example of synaesthesia in the combining of the senses of hearing and seeing. Their synaesthesia combines the senses of seeing and touching/feeling for super empaths, so that if they can see another person being physically touched, then they can feel it in their own body too. The researchers also found that the people who witnessed this "mirror-touch" phenomenon were also more likely to display high levels of emotional empath, drawing on very subtle energies and emotions. This illustrates how the neural roles of the empath make them even more sensitive to picking up on and even internalizing other people's feelings, so much so that they could even feel touched by another person.

By recognizing the way empath operates inside the human brain, we are able to learn more about empath itself. Empaths experience the same empathic neural mechanisms as others, but they are simply more responsive and experience these processes to a greater extent in general. We are able to better understand why we are the way we are, and how we can better improve our empath in a way that best benefits us and those around us by distinguishing between the various neural mechanisms that tell our personalities and behaviors.

CHAPTER 4:

EMPATHS – THE GOOD, THE BAD AND THE UGLY

Now that some of the characteristics of empaths have been identified, we can discuss how becoming an empath can affect the life of an individual. Empaths, as has already been developed, have different levels of sensitivity towards different stimulants, particularly in social settings. That isn't always a bad thing though. This only means that they appear to be more introverted and prefer to relax after social encounters by spending time alone. Much like any form of personality, empath is not one-size-fits-all. There are many different characteristics that contribute to empaths, and to different degrees, many people experience different traits.

Now let's explore the ways it can be immensely helpful to identify as empath, as well as the difficulties that the empath sometimes faces. On many occasions, empaths can also encounter many behaviors, thus discovering that different attributes do not necessarily relate to their particular circumstances. There are also various situations in an individual that can bring out different traits. You will note when you find yourself being distant or being overwhelmed by stimuli by knowing your empathetic characteristics. Major changes can also cause this to happen, so you can remain focused and prioritize self-care by understanding your empathic qualities. It is important to note that forms and characteristics of personalities are highly complex. One attribute can one day appear as a gift, and the next as a curse.

In addition, personalities are complex and can alter and grow depending on various factors such as your climate, the people you associate yourself with, and your education. Therefore, depending on these variables, many of the characteristics that empaths acquire vary, and these basic characteristics may end up working entirely different, based on the individual and their circumstances. For example, while one individual may love their hypersensitivity because it enables them to develop deeper emotional bonds with other individuals, another individual may find that their hypersensitivity causes them to become frustrated and isolate themselves from other individuals.

This example shows how one common personality trait, depending on the individual, may have the opposite effect. With this in mind, in combination with your other attributes, you will determine the qualities you possess and how they manifest in your everyday life. You will be better able to determine how you identify as an empath, by looking at the pieces and the whole of your personality, and you will learn more about yourself and your personal skills, as well as the difficulties you can face.

BENEFITS OF BEING AN EMPATH

Most of what we see as advantages of identifying as empath lies behind those inconsistencies. Although an empath would possibly consider itself an introvert, many of its gifts often lie in being a people person. Since empaths are able to absorb other people's feelings and energies around them, they are naturally very good at reading people. This also means they have good intuition and instincts in general, which can prove to be a very practical life ability. This is useful in that they are excellent at selecting who is trustworthy and who is dishonest.

Although these abilities can often seem daunting, being a strong character judge is certainly a big help for empaths. This insight and character judgment can not come as naturally with non-empaths who have issues connected to other individuals, which can trigger problems. Empaths can also tell when a person is lying to them, which can prove to be an important skill in contemporary society. In various careers that work with other individuals, these talents also help them succeed. Empaths also make excellent teachers, therapists, health care professionals, business people, and every other position requiring a deep understanding of individuals. Being a good human behavior predictor is one of the strongest qualities of an empath.

Empaths are also excellent at defending themselves and others from intimidating individuals because they have sound judgment and instincts. Did you ever meet someone you felt was just a little off? Perhaps it was the new significant other of your friend who had dubious motives, and you proved right. This is a basic functional capacity that an empath possesses, and that possibly goes back to empath's evolutionary origins. The capacity of empaths to experience energy and feelings helps them recognize threats quickly, and defend themselves and those around them. Another advantage of their gift of deep and precise insight is this. If you think you have strong instincts and your first instinct is typically right, but your abilities have not been completely established, then you might still be an empath. Many empaths have intuition, but since they have not formed it, it is dormant. In addition, this powerful insight, such as manifestation or lucid dreaming, can be used for several different gifts. In the next chapter, we'll concentrate on how you can discover your natural abilities and grow them.

Empaths are normally very innovative people as well. This is one of the gifts that come with an empathic personality that can be built and honed, but usually, empaths feel that they naturally come to creativity. They can turn these feelings into artistic expressions, such as art, because empaths are so in contact with emotions and sensitive to different emotions. Although individuals who are closed off and disconnected from their feelings can have trouble with creative blocks, empaths can normally channel and convey their feelings naturally. Not only can they do so by tapping into their own emotions, but because they can so quickly absorb other people's emotions, they can even transmit other people's emotions.

This imagination, such as painting, literature, or even different spiritual practices, can translate into many distinct forms. Channeling the emotions of others makes empaths understanding to the point of expression, which is a creative asset. Moreover, this imagination will allow empaths to better explore the energy that flows inside and without humans. Empaths can better understand their own inner energies through artistic writing, which can improve both the self-expression and self-understanding. By consuming and channeling the emotions of other cultures, empaths will, in fact, become more in tune with their own thoughts and feelings.

The capacity to heal others is another gift that empaths possess. Since they can recognize, understand, experience, and act upon other people's feelings, this makes them really able to determine how to support people. This is one of the attributes that makes such strong therapists and doctors feel empathic. Empath, though, also makes perfect holistic doctors and energy healers, because they are so much in tune with the energy that others are projecting. Empaths may also feel as if they are curing themselves by curing others. If you identify as empath, then in several group settings, you probably find yourself taking on the role of mediator.

Do you find yourself feeling happier as a result when you support friends or family? This is because, when there's a problem, you internalize the negative energy. If your friends are battling, even if you are not directly involved, as a consequence of all the negativity and misery swirling around you, you can feel irritated and nervous. However, by acting as a mediator, you can heal the energy which negatively affects both your friends and you. This also benefits you, in a way, as you boost the vibrations that surround you, helping you to internalize more positive emotions.

This is a major reason why empaths use their healing gift, so they can heal themselves by healing others too. This shows the altruistic nature of empath. Empaths want to assist others because they feel better because of it. This is also why in professions where they support people, such as in nursing or therapy, empaths are also able to feel incredibly fulfilled.

Empaths also have the unusual ability to build deep bonds with other people and cultivate them. This can be incredibly rewarding, as they find that in their lives they have the potential to develop very close relationships with people. Interestingly enough, in addition to humans, the empath may also shape those deep bonds with animals. They are able to perceive the feelings of other species, and they have a deep connection with nature as well. As it offers satisfaction, this caring capacity to build relationships with various individuals and even animals is a gift to empath. Though introverted, Empaths ultimately desire communication. Since they are so capable of consuming energy and feelings, they can create these bonds quickly, which contributes to emotional fulfillment. This makes good partners, friends, and family members feel empathetic.

Ultimately, possessing these powerful emotional skills and the ability to build strong emotional connections helps empaths to draw tons of love and positivity into their lives. In addition, while experiencing the pain and sorrow of others can seem like a downside of being an empath, they still feel the pleasure and affection of other people. Essentially, they feel it in a heightened way as empaths feel joy, which is one of their greatest gifts. These are all gifts that allow empaths with other people to build powerful and unique emotional connections. These connections also enable them to excel in various aspects of their lives, especially in interpersonal situations. Empaths are very well-liked in general, making them good friends, partners, co-workers, etc. In social settings, this helps them feel relaxed and valued, which can in turn put them more at ease in the case of overstimulation. This is one of the greatest gifts that come with being an empath, and these strong bonds are also reinforced by some of the setbacks that empath could face.

CHALLENGES OF BEING AN EMPATH AND HOW TO OVERCOME THEM

Although becoming an empath is definitely a gift valued by many people, it does come with its fair share of challenges. If you identify as empath, then you may be faced with all of these problems even if you have not officially classified or even identified them. Whether or not you feel that you are susceptible to any of the characteristics mentioned, acknowledging them is important to understand how to cope with some of the external difficulties resulting from being an empath. In addition, you might see an overlap between some of these common challenges and many of the gifts we just went through that you have.

This is because, depending on the setting, many of the characteristics the empath possesses may be positive or bad. In the past, you would not have given this much thought. But you can recognize how they both negatively and positively impact your life by identifying these attributes now, and how you can become more in tune with yourself. As an empath, you are possibly very attuned to other people's emotions and resources.

But this book will help you become more in tune with yourself by teaching you about what makes you. Overstimulation is a common challenge faced by empath, as already stated as a characteristic of empath. Since their brains are basically hypersensitive to distinct stimuli, in situations where they are surrounded by a lot of people and/or movement, empaths may quickly become overwhelmed and exhausted. Particularly in circumstances, empaths can experience this even with people they are close to, simply because they need time to recharge alone. This may have been experienced in a school or workplace environment. Has a friend ever asked you to grab dinner after work but after 8 hours of intense stimulation, you just couldn't imagine spending any more time with other people? This is nothing to be ashamed of—it just means you're recharging by spending time on your own.

There are some steps you should take to prevent the consequences of overstimulation if you are in a career or living condition that allows you to be constantly surrounded by other individuals. Self-care is extremely necessary, particularly for empaths (which we will address in later chapters), to ensure that we allow ourselves to recover from over-stimulation and burnout. Another thing empaths may do to integrate some time alone to recover is to take breaks or maintain some kind of distance. If you live with roommates, and feel like you're constantly surrounded by people, locking yourself in your room for some time alone is perfect. As no one wants to spend time with someone who is obviously tired and not themselves, people are normally really understanding.

The overload of negative energy is another problem that empathizers often face in their daily lives. This can be in any situation, but if you're surrounded by negative people who can't stop moaning, or you're also getting irritated after checking out the news, it's probably a sign that you need some self-care. We will also concentrate on later chapters on energy healing for empaths. Since empaths are so easily able to absorb even the most subtle energy around them, they could find themselves exhausted or emotionally distracted as a consequence if they are around many negative people. It is very important to practice self-care, energy healing, and solitary activities to prevent the overwhelming feeling.

You will also find that you need to spend less time with the people who drain your energy from you or make you feel negative feelings while you are around them. This is also a form of self-care—it is important to cut constantly negative people out of your life, particularly for empath, to protect and ensure your own happiness. This is better said than done, of course, and another obstacle posed by an empath is that they appear to attract these negative individuals. This is the book for you if you feel as if you are constantly pulling adverse energy into your life and have no idea how to stop, particularly in social situations. The first step is to recognize that you might be sensitive to these traits. When you begin to notice who and what continually triggers you to experience negative feelings or to be drained mentally, you will start to find out when you can recover.

ANOTHER SIDE EFFECT THAT EMPATHS FACE IS A TRAIT THAT WAS MENTIONED EARLIER: LONELINESS

This is another inconsistency empath offers us, as one would think an empath is an individual of the people. Loneliness, however, may be prevalent among empaths, especially those who, when they become frustrated and exhausted, isolate themselves from other people. To the point of distance, a typical setback of being an empath is being overwhelmed. There is a fine line between taking time alone to refresh and distancing yourself so often so that you become lonely, and this can sometimes be struggling when stimulation is strong.

Empaths can also find that due to the struggle of continuous overstimulation, they scare people away in close relationships. This can lead to solitude, and a feeling other people don't understand. Another feature of empath that can contribute to loneliness is their insight into the characters of others. This can result in them posing as judgmental or standoffish, which can be off-putting to others. Ultimately, however, this is a positive attribute, because it helps you to make sure that the people in your life are positive for you. It also encourages you to create relationships on actual interactions rather than just commonalities at the surface level, which is inherently beneficial. However, there are steps you should take to stop distancing yourself from others if you want to focus on this simply to make a stronger first impression.

The increased vulnerability to mental illness may be another potential negative side effect of being an empath. Empaths are also diagnosed with social anxiety, or misdiagnosed, because of their propensity to feel distracted and nervous in certain people's environments. Empaths are often more likely than normal to experience other psychiatric problems as a result of trying to cope with overstimulation, such as depression or drug use disorders.

Empaths may be at risk of developing drug use disorders as a way to try to avoid the overstimulation they may face, according to Dr. Orloff's study. Since empaths are simply "sponges" to the emotions of other people, being surrounded by too much negative energy will make them more likely to develop an addiction to a drug. Drugs and alcohol often numb or distract from the heightened stimuli encountered by an empath's hypersensitive brain, making them dependent on those substances.

Empaths are often susceptible to anxiety, depression, and other problems simply because they are hypersensitive to their brains. While certain unpleasant experiences can be shrugged off by a non-empath, empaths don't have the same capacity to do so. This can result in multiple conditions being formed. Empaths, however, are able to establish and practice secure coping strategies through adequate care and treatment. This is why being self-aware and staying in touch with your inner self is extremely necessary. It would be very helpful in the long run to identify your behavior patterns and know when to seek help, since you will be able to recognize whether you have an addictive attitude and/or a vulnerability to any mental illnesses.

With respect to their sensitivity and kindness, there are also other obstacles that empaths face. Although these are positive things, empaths will also feel as though they are being manipulated by other people. Empaths are instinctively loving and compassionate people, which can cause them to attract people who benefit from their empath and drain their energy in essence. It is also sometimes said that empaths are "too sensitive," which can contribute to awkward interactions. This can also create problems with establishing relationships with other people, particularly in early life. In school settings, empaths will also face challenges, as they also learn how to cope with their empathic behaviors while still learning how to develop new relationships with other individuals.

Empaths are not unusual to face difficulty making friends, especially in large groups, because of how hypersensitive they are. They're also vulnerable to boundary setting difficulties. Since empaths are so caring and want to support people with their feelings, they can be taken advantage of this in a different way. People can cross borders, and expect too much from empath. Empaths, therefore, also find themselves unable to say "no," physically and emotionally exhausted and feeling taken-for-granted. They may also feel as if they are attracting people who take advantage of them in this regard, which may lead to them getting into toxic relationships consistently. Ultimately, this is also because empaths also crave the feeling of helping others and want to feel as if they care about others. This can, however, result in unhealthy relationships and bad habits.

This is why it is a form of self-care to learn to set boundaries. By establishing limits, empaths will ensure that they no longer feel as though they are taken for granted by the people around them. Also, it can avoid mental burnout. Last but not least, empaths will battle self-care. Despite this being extremely necessary to recharge, empaths also put the interests of others before their own. This can be dangerous behavior, since neglecting your own emotions can end up having a detrimental effect on your relationships with others. You can discover that you can be a stronger version of your empathic self by giving priority to your own mental and emotional well-being.

CHAPTER 5:

TOOLS FOR TRANSFORMATION AND SPIRITUAL GROWTH

As we described earlier, the empath has several competencies linked to various spiritual traditions. Typically, empaths are very in touch with energy and intuition, making them likely to have clairvoyant or intuitive skills. But even if you don't think you're psychic, your empathic abilities may make you more likely to believe in various spiritual processes such as healing energy, manifestation, balancing chakras, and meditation. Although there are a lot of different spiritual processes that empaths may find gravitating toward, we will concentrate more generally on spirituality in general.

Western culture does not generally provide us with a large range of resources to build a lifestyle with our intuitive gifts. So many of us probably aren't even conscious of these talents we hold. A lot of spirituality can also be written off as "mumbo jumbo" that concerns energy cycles and the intuition of an individual. However, one of their biggest abilities is an empath's intuition, and learning how to tap into it is a perfect way to become more in tune with your feelings and flows of energy.

This will then help you communicate with others more, and you will see the advantages of learning how to manage your own energy flows more. If you've ever felt like witnessing any strange coincidences or deja vu often, this could be an unconscious illustration of your inner intuition at work. You might not know it, but inside of you, your intuition may still be powerful, but it has just been suppressed. However, even if you don't feel as if you have a good natural intuition, you can still build and strive to strengthen these skills. When we explore how we should work to improve our talents, let's first dig into what spirituality is and how the empath relates to it.

WHAT IS SPIRITUALITY?

There is no single simple concept of spirituality, particularly because it covers such a large part of human experience and can be applied to many different aspects of life. Spirituality can generally be described as the relation between a human being and what they believe to be a greater being or mechanism. Spirituality is also called finding intent or meaning. This quest may take place inside the human body and spirit, or without it. Spirituality, however, is a simple and age-old facet of human life. It primarily refers to our feelings of connectedness and intention, and by looking inward, we can also learn more about our personal beliefs.

Some people in faith feel this bond and engage in worship to feel the bond to a higher being. Some people consider the universe idea to be an underlying being, and prefer to engage in various activities that bind them to the universe, such as manifestation or meditation. Some individuals claim that by tuning in to our own energies, we can relate to this greater being. This is where intuition comes into play, and in order to regulate and track our own energy flows and processes, we will concentrate primarily on this part of our spirituality. It is important to remember that there is no straight cut to how we convey our spirituality. In a religious context, one should believe in a higher force, but at the same time believing that they are an empath with a deep intuition and the ability to draw on the energy of others.

You may learn something based on your own unique energies and processes, but you want to express your spirituality. Spirituality, though often a communal experience, is really just about having your personal connection to whatever higher force you trust. This means that you concentrate your energies inward to tap into your energy source and build that bond with whatever higher force you try to connect to. By communicating with your own instincts, you will find out a lot about yourself, your energy, and the world around you. This natural intuition is probably already powerful as an empath, which will allow you to really tap into your source of energy and build those powerful flows between yourself and the higher power.

Seven criteria were established by psychological researcher Howard Clinebell that humans frequently apply to their quest for meaning. In their practice of spirituality, these requirements are what they always look for. Clinebell determined that mind, body, spirit, love, play, and the world are the 7 requirements that he presented in a 1992 novel. We look for love, for example, whether it is in ourselves or with others. This is something that empaths also have as a primary focus, as they ultimately want to feel the love they can feel so sensitively and offer so freely. However, instead of looking inward, where empaths may go wrong in their spiritual journey is in their outward quest for love. Empaths can find a good balance by being more in tune with their own feelings, so as to find satisfaction inside and not feel like they have to look for it in someone else.

Human beings often pursue something greater than themselves naturally, seeking to establish a connection. Without even noticing it, this is something that empaths sometimes do. By tuning in and knowing the energies of other people, they can sense a connection outside themselves. These are only a few examples of how sometimes, without even understanding it, empaths create a spiritual bond. These requirements are basically the forms in which spirituality always looks for fulfillment. For example, we may seek fulfillment through physical movement; several exercises, like yoga, function as spiritual acts, as linking our body to a higher force helps us to feel in control and enables us to elevate our energetic vibrations.

On an abstract level, we still search for fulfillment when it applies to the mind. We aspire to improve our comprehension and our ability to enhance our analytical skills. Through these various parameters, as we pursue fulfillment in our lives, we find ourselves seeking an energetic and spiritual connection.

Empaths may also feel that they need spiritual therapy to move beyond their need for fulfillment and connection. Dr. Orloff, who is not only an empath but has done comprehensive studies on empath, has coined the concept "energy psychiatry" as a mean of combining spirituality with the conventional practice of medical treatment to healing the mind, body, and spirit. In order to use subtle energy as a means of healing, this technique was created. This enables us to tap into our energetic strength, which Orloff often claims is made to lie dormant. In order to create a greater link with our spirit and the world and energies around us, this idea illustrates how we can use various aspects of spirituality.

Orloff explicitly addresses the advantages of such activities as meditation and Reiki energy healing, which are also considered complementary types of medicine. Additionally, Orloff cites the importance of intuition in healing, saying that intuition will improve inner guidance. Since empaths naturally have a powerful intuition, they will find that they are able to look inward in healing by using various spiritual practices to enhance this gift. In addition, in cultivating one's own intuition, patients can potentially be more beneficial to physicians and healers. This again relates to the ways empaths are intrinsically good healers, and can help others. An individual can pick up on all the subtle energies that flow inside and beyond the body by establishing a close link with one's own mind and body.

Essentially, we will find that many of the answers to the questions we seek lie within us by reinforcing the inner mechanism of intuition. This, for example, connects in processes such as manifestation and meditation. Both of these spiritual processes demand that we look inward to establish our spiritual relations. Empaths are also very experienced at harnessing energy using their intuition, precisely because they are able to pick up on subtle energy flows. This makes it very easy for empaths to use their spiritual gifts, even without thinking about it consciously. Empaths are capable of picking up on energetic vibrations naturally.

When applying this to behavior such as manifestation and actually channeling the energies they can pick up on, they are usually very good at understanding what they need and how to attract it. In the next pages, we will explore how empaths can function and apply them to spiritual processes to improve their skills of intuition. But let's start by defining a few terms and explaining some processes first. Your intuition refers to your innate ability, not logic or reasoning, to grasp something purely based on implicit instinct. You certainly have a good intuition as an empath, whether you ever acknowledge it consciously, or not. Have you ever experienced a moment where they ordered you to do one thing, but you had a feeling of gut urging you to do another? At work, this is your intuition. This also shows how empath can be an ability for survival. By possessing these powerful, intuitive abilities, humans can defend themselves and their lives. It also helps you to be a good character judge, which is a highly useful ability in life.

One way that many people contact their intuition is by dreaming. Empaths are known for having extremely vivid dreams as very imaginative and intuitive people. These dreams will give them insight and clarity into the world's own perceptions. The feeling that things that occur in their dreams come true in real life is a common phenomenon that empaths can experience. This in your mind is your intuition at work, even though you're unconscious. Today, this does not actually apply to being able to predict major events such as an earthquake or a stock market crash (although some people claim to be able to do this), but rather less predictable events that occur in daily life. Have you ever developed a sense of deja vu while doing something totally random, like sitting in class or commuting to work? At work, this is your intuition. Although this may sound like it's just a random thought, there are actually ways to tap your intuition as it appears in your dreams.

In the next sections we will get into strategies but another way to see your intuition played out in your dreams is by lucid dreaming. Lucid dreaming is a phenomenon that is not completely understood by humans while studied by researchers. In essence, when you are unconscious and dreaming, a lucid dream is, however you are consciously aware that what happens in your dream is not true. This effectively puts you in charge of your dream, allowing you to be the film director and not just a cast member. When you have a very vivid dream, lucid dreaming takes place, but you are aware that the events that occur in your dream are not actual, which distinguishes your conscious mind from your unconscious mind in a way.

Have you ever had a nightmare and then find yourself thinking, while still having the dream, 'This is not real?' This is a genuinely lucid dreaming example. Lucid dreaming can give us a sense of control which we can take into our daily lives. We may also tap into our intuition by influencing how it is conveyed by studying the lucid dream. Lucid dreaming can also be used as a kind of treatment for people with recurring nightmares. Even if you don't always find yourself having these kinds of dreams, but you want to see if your unconscious intuition can begin to be managed, there are techniques that help you to improve your ability to dream lucidly.

Another way you can connect to your instincts is by meditation practice. Meditation is an age-old activity of sitting with your thoughts and watching them, allowing them to flow freely and also concentrating on your breath as you do. But this concept is extremely wide, and there are innumerable ways and types of meditation. Meditation is simply a way to communicate with your inner energies and instincts by allowing your brain to observe the unconscious and to get in contact with it. Meditation, either in combination with other rituals or by itself, is also used as a spiritual activity and can also be used in counseling and holistic medical treatments. Meditation has many proven advantages, and empaths should explicitly meditate to re-equilibrate their resources and recover after long periods of social contact.

There are numerous types of meditation, too, but the main ones are concentrated meditation and free meditation. You concentrate on something in concentrated meditation, whether it is on the rhythm of your breath or directed meditation. This helps you to focus your mind on something so that you can stop wondering about it. However, free forms of meditation encourage you just to let your thoughts flow in and out. You don't really concentrate on something but you just note and release your thoughts. For empaths, this is a perfect way to start grounding themselves. You can find that by meditating and observing your emotions, then releasing them without responding to them, you will exercise control over what you let affect you and what you respond to. In your daily life, this will then encourage you to practice this power, and you will find it much easier to avoid the energies of other people from influencing you so profoundly.

The idea of manifestation is another spiritual phenomenon that is also related to dreaming, intuition, and meditation. Manifestation is a practice that incorporates the laws of energy and the universe and focuses fundamentally on the premise that the energy we project is the energy that will come to us. In the fields of self-help and spirituality, this approach has recently become very popular and is often used in combination with meditation. There are also such strategies and methods that indicate that in your dreams you will manifest yourself. Whatever the case, when performed by a highly intuitive person, manifestation is always incredibly effective simply because it takes intense concentration, and in order to function, you need to be very clear and precise about the emotions that will emerge from something you manifest.

We will get into manifestation strategies in the next section that prove to be especially useful for empath. In order to function, this method uses the Law of Attraction. The Law of Attraction is a law of energy that states that what we attract is the energy we put out. For example, if you genuinely believe that you're going to have a good day, and continue to reiterate that to yourself during the day, you're going to concentrate on the positive things that happen to you, and you're going to have a good day most likely. If you keep thinking and talking negatively, though, telling yourself that you're going to have a bad day, you're going to definitely have a bad day. This is because what we are drawing back into our lives is the energy that we bring out into the world. In addition, when we concentrate on a single thought or concept, that's what we'll find in our lives. This will still sound a little confusing, so in the next part, we will get into this practice.

DEVELOPING YOUR INTUITION

If you are fascinated by some of these processes, but you still do not fully understand how to make spirituality work in your daily life, then look no further than this book. In order to cultivate your intuition and apply it to various spiritual and therapeutic practices, there are many ways that you can tap into yourself and others' feelings. One common method at which empaths are especially skilled is energy healing, which we will address in the next chapter in-depth.

However, there are many things that require practice and technique to create, despite natural gifts that make empaths trained in various processes that convey their intuition. Remember that spirituality is a journey—it may seem daunting at first to practice harnessing your instincts and energy, but you'll find out what's right for you as you go on. You will also become more in tune with your own feelings and energies, which will teach you how to be more in equilibrium with both yourself and the greater force you believe in. The best way of harnessing the energies into a spiritual path and seeking fulfillment is to achieve inner peace. You will find yourself reflecting on gratitude and the good aspects of your life as you tap into this stream of energy, preserving this energy in turn.

You've just read about what lucid dreaming is, for example, and you might now wonder to yourself how people do this often, and how they can use it to make their lives easier. If you'd like to learn how to dream lucidly but don't know where to start, here are some tips. Practice checking your truth is one way to begin lucid dreaming. You also find yourself being overstimulated by your brain as an empath, which can cause you to get enveloped in your thoughts. You can start by grounding yourself, if you notice this occurring during the day. Try to "test" your truth by asking yourself if real life is really what is happening around you. By doing this, when you are awake and feel caught up in your thoughts, your brain will know, when unconscious, how to go through these motions. Then, ideally, in your sleep, you will be able to do this, reminding yourself to verify your reality even while you are unconscious and dreaming.

Another technique that will help you with your lucid dream is to wake up in the middle of the night and then return to sleep. People also do this if they wake up unexpectedly in the middle of the night, but if you set an alarm to wake up deliberately, remember your surroundings consciously, and the fact that you are awake and then go back to sleep, you might find it easier to feel in control of your dreams. Keeping a dream journal in which you record your dreams when you first wake up is another technique that helps with lucid dreaming, and with tracking your dreams in general. Throughout the day, many people forget their dreams, so remembering them as soon as you wake up when they're still fresh in your mind is a good way to recall the feelings that happened in your dreams. This is also a good way to keep track of any patterns or predictions that occur in your dreams, and it can be a good way for empaths to note their thoughts and their subconscious representation of them. Keeping in contact with the unconscious self is a perfect way for empaths to feel a connection to the source of their inner energies.

Meditation is another spiritual activity that involves some technique and repetition. As we have already learned, there are many different ways of meditation. You could want to do a guided meditation or just sit down and watch your breath patterns. You might meditate with manifesting intention, or you might want to heal your energies and align your chakras. Whatever the case, many individuals also fail to be still and to observe their own feelings and thoughts. This can present a challenge, in particular for empaths, simply because empaths also have active minds and are overwhelmed with emotions and stimuli. However, if you are able to step beyond these distractions, if you feel stressed or exhausted, you will find that meditating is a perfect way to ground yourself and refresh.

It is necessary to bear in mind that there are multiple meditation methods, and there is not one that is better than the other. It's important to figure out what works best for you, instead. For example, when concentrating on one particular thing, such as your breath, you might choose to meditate. This is a good route for many empaths, as it gives you a more sense of power. It will prevent your mind from wandering too far, enabling you to really relax. It also helps to anchor you, and if you feel overwhelmed by your emotions, concentrating on your breath allows you to come back to the practice of meditation. But you don't have to concentrate on the inhalation and exhalation process while you meditate. You might actually choose to observe the thoughts that are crossing your mind, and then just let them go. This may also be a perfect empath tool, as it helps you to observe the resources and feelings that take up a great deal of room in your mind.

However, if you sometimes get overstimulated and find your mind wandering, this strategy can be difficult. This is because you simply need to remember a thought, whether it's about your world or something happening in your life, and then just let it go without answering or worrying about it. It takes practice to release your thoughts in this way, as empaths are susceptible to overthinking. This is why a good way to begin meditating is always to concentrate on your breath. In the end, this will stabilize your feelings and help you become more in contact with your feelings. Also, you can try guided meditations, usually created in the form of videos in which a narrator talks and informs you what to concentrate on. This can be another great way to start meditating and can be great if you are considering meditating for a certain target. This can be a strong manifesting tool, as well.

Another excellent way to channel your innate intuition is through manifestation. This is also achieved with meditation, as meditation before and after you manifest enhances insight and helps you to really get what you need to tap into your inner source of energy. Although manifestation is obviously a very complicated process, and there isn't necessarily a "right" way to do it, we'll provide a quick guide on how you can start manifesting in your own life. Naturally the first step in manifestation is to determine explicitly what you want to manifest and attract. Empaths are fortunate that their innate intelligence helps them to see clearly what they need and want to pull into their lives.

Focusing on the feelings associated with what you are manifesting is important—you might even only be manifesting a feeling in your life itself, like more happiness or affection. Visualizing what you are attempting to manifest is critical then. Empaths are also skilled at doing this because their intuition helps them to be very imaginative and visualizing very well. Visualization is an important step in manifestation, as it's important to build the feelings you'll have when you've expressed what you want. In essence, you must assume that you already have what it is that you are seeking to attract. In order to make your visualization more successful, this is a method that you can do through meditation, or even lucid dreaming.

It is important to release the thought after you've visualized it. Don't dwell on what you want but don't have, because dwelling on this shortage would only draw more shortages.

Live your life with the illusion you've got what you want, instead. You may also take steps, while also bringing this feeling, to accomplish what you want. For example, if you want to draw more love into your life, show appreciation for all the love you have at the moment. Love yourself, then, and add all this love to your own spirit and the important relationships you have. You'll be able to draw more of them by showing appreciation for all the positive things you already have in your life.

CHAPTER 6:

EMPATHS AND ENERGY

We've briefly discussed the idea of energy healing in the last few chapters, and how empaths are usually very much in tune with the energy of both themselves and others, but now we're going to really dive into the idea of energy. Energy is a driving force of life, and all kinds of things can be interpreted utilizing it. Biologically, energy is what holds and drives us alive. We can, however, look at the word "power" in its spiritual context in order to explain the way that empaths function on a spiritual basis. Like many of the other definitions we have described so far, energy can apply to a lot of different processes and definitions and be applied to them. The term "power," though, typically refers to the inner root of anyone. People may sometimes refer to energy as one's spirit, aura, or "vibe." The "energy" of an individual is often related to it and refers to its inner power. If you've ever heard someone say they don't like the energy of a person, it can mean they feel like it isn't matched with their own. Sometimes we can also internalize negativity around us, causing it to cloud our focus. This can make us more cynical, in turn.

Empaths are particularly vulnerable to these actions because they internalize so much of the energy around them. Energy flows continually all over us, and this is also particularly visible for empath. Although we do not all think consciously of the energies around us, empaths do find that this has an implicit influence on what they do. For example, if you've ever been to a library during the final week, after you left, you've probably found yourself feeling much more nervous than when you came into the library. This is because all the nervous energy around you has been internalized by you. This also extends to empaths, which is why spending lots of time in social environments, particularly crowds, can be so difficult for them. Energy healing is an age-old method, and it may be his own book to describe the way energy functions in a spiritual context. We can start by illustrating various belief systems that concentrate on energy healing for the purposes of clarification. The theory of chakras is one principle of energy that is applied to several different activities, such as yoga, energy healing, acupuncture, and meditation. The term "chakra" is a Sanskrit word, which refers to one's energy source. In many Hindu and Buddhist traditions, chakras are central to various practices. There are 7 chakras, and each is a source of energy in the body that focuses on various parts of the life of an individual. It is believed that the energy of an individual flows inside and without their chakras, and that energy can become blocked in one or more chakras, which in one's life can cause negative effects. In order to resolve this, aligned chakras need to be preserved, and any energy blockages removed. Depending on the chakra, this can also be done by yoga, meditation, or numerous individual activities. Later in this chapter, we will discuss common locations that are unique to empath to remedy blockage. But we'll outline each of the chakras first.

ROOT CHAKRA

The root chakra is referred to as the first chakra, and at the base of the spine it can be found. It is connected to the color red and to the grounding, protection, base, and security functions. A feeling that you lack equilibrium, a sense of loneliness, or fear may be indicators of an imbalance of the root chakra. This may be a common issue facing empath, as they can quickly become frustrated by change and overstimulation. It is important to ground yourself when this occurs. By engaging in relaxing practices, including self-reflection, spending time in nature, and remaining in a relaxed environment, the root chakra can be unblocked. Through meditation and yoga we can heal the root chakra too.

HOLY CHAKRA

The second chakra is the sacral chakra, in the pelvic area. The color orange and the roles of enjoyment, intimacy, and imagination are associated with it. As they are inherently intuitive and imaginative, many empaths will discover that it is easy for them to align their sacral chakras. In the sacral chakra, symptoms of an imbalance may be issues with intimacy and communicating feelings and trouble communicating passion. By participating in artistic practices, coping with pent-up feelings, yoga, and meditation, the sacral chakra may be unblocked. This often sometimes happens when empaths have relationship trouble or are unable to communicate their feelings. Loading up and taking time alone to note your feelings is a perfect way to unblock this chakra.

SOLAR PLEXUS CHAKRA

The third chakra is the Chakra of the solar plexus, also known as the Manipura. She is in the stomach. It is related to the yellow color and relates to several inner functions, such as self-esteem, trust, and motivation. This can be a common source of energy blockage for empaths, since they derive a lot of their energy from that of others. Signs of an imbalance in this chakra include a loss of self-confidence and motivation. Through yoga the Manipura can be unblocked, meditation to tap into your inner intent, and goal planning. If you find yourself struggling with your Manipura, rather than relying on other people's, make sure to tap into your own inner root and explore your own emotions.

THE HEART CHAKRA

The heart chakra, positioned around the heart and lungs, is the fourth chakra. This chakra, associated with the color green, is connected with both inner and outer love and compassion. Signs that this chakra is blocked include lack of self-respect, problems with other people's relationships, and denial of respect. For empaths, the heart chakra is an incredibly common source of energy blockage. A lack of self-love can result from closing off or internalizing too much negative energy, which may influence relationships in turn. You can notice, however, that your heart chakra is rather overactive, as an empath. You may find yourself, as someone who is profoundly linked to other people, putting so much energy into others yet neglecting your own self. This can lead to insecurity and low self-esteem, which is why learning how to put yourself first is extremely important. By meditation, yoga, and practicing self-love by affirmations, this chakra can be unblocked.

THE THROAT CHAKRA

The fifth chakra is the chakra of the throat connected to the blue hue. Its functions include speech, language, and communication. Obviously, Empaths care deeply for the feelings of others, even putting them above their own.

Also, they are susceptible to attracting people who suck their resources. As a consequence, they might feel as though they are being spoken about endlessly or that their desires and interests are being placed under those of other people. A blocked chakra of the throat is characterized by an inability to communicate thoughts and feelings and communication difficulties. Through meditation, affirmations, breathwork, and journaling, this chakra can be unblocked.

THE THIRD EYE CHAKRA

The sixth chakra is the chakra of the third eye, positioned in between the eyes. It is associated with the purple color and intuition and interior reflection functions. Empaths, on account of their deep intuition, usually have a very open and active third-eye chakra. But even empaths may experience blockages here, particularly if they have suppressed or enabled their natural intuitive gifts to dorm. A blocked third-eye chakra is characterized by a lack of simple intuition and a sense of disconnection from your inner self. Even if you have good empathic instincts, you can feel detached from your own feelings, since you are so focused on other people's emotions. It is possible to unblock this chakra through time alone, self-reflection, and meditation.

THE CROWN CHAKRA

The crown chakra, positioned right at the top of the head, is the last chakra. The color white is associated with this chakra, and it focuses on the movement of energy in our outer world. This works to link our inner flows of energy with the outer world. By tapping into our inner source of energy, we will interact with the world that is around us. Empaths in this regard are inherently talented, since they are very much in tune with the energies flowing around them. A blocked crown chakra can manifest in the form of close-mindedness or a sense of disconnection in the universe around you. This chakra can be unblocked for reconnecting with the outer world by means of meditation, yoga, and affirmations. Understanding how different chakras dictate energy flows in different regions of the body helps us focus on balancing different aspects of our lives. Through knowing the way energy in the chakras can become blocked or even overactive, we can even gain insight into the physical illnesses that occur in various parts of the body. Since discussing some of the ways our energy flows, we can now look into how this applies directly to empaths.

HOW DO EMPATHS AFFECT ENERGY FLOWS?

Since empaths can actually sense the feelings of another person so quickly, they also pick up on the energy flows of other people. This may mean, however, that if they don't pay attention, they can mistake the energy of another person for their own. For example, an empath may find themselves feeling stressed out by spending a lot of time with a particularly nervous individual. It can then be difficult to discern whether this feeling of fear is their own, or whether it is the nervous energy they pick up from another person instead.

Empaths, in this sense, would appear to boost whatever energy they pick up on, whether good or bad. They will serve as a kind of catalyst for the energy being projected around them—internalizing it and then, in exchange, projecting more of the same energy. This can be a good thing too if an empath can ground itself and learn how to channel positive energy. When they are able to project the positive energy they have internalized, the vibrations around them can be lifted in turn. This is why people are always so drawn to empath; when they are around them, they put them in a good mood, and this allows for strong relationships.

Empaths often appear to pick up on all the energy that affects them, even though it is normally undesirable. They think of energy as a common being and something exchanged by various spirits. Although certain non-empaths are good at shielding their energy and are usually unfazed by what happens to other individuals, to do this, empaths are often too sensitive. Rather, they are evidently unable to block the stimulators around them, with many of those stimulators being the patterns of energy they pick up on. This energy is then likely to be internalized by them. It is important to note that energy blockages within our bodies can also be pent up, causing imbalances in various aspects of our lives. Setting boundaries is important, particularly for empaths. Not only will this allow you to protect your emotions and refresh, but you will also protect your energy from internalizing any harmful vibrations by establishing boundaries. Getting energy bottled up or blocked can also impact our physical health. Different chakras control different parts of the body, and the chakras are correlated with different physical ailments.

The theory of energy meridians, close to chakras, is another energy principle.

Meridians are sometimes used in Chinese medicine, and it is believed that there is a sort of linked pathway that flows across the body from various energy sources. In each organ, these meridians concentrate and form a kind of map for our energy to flow through our bodies. Not only do the meridians perform biological functions and sustain homeostasis in our bodies, but they also provide a free energy flow. This helps our 'chi' or 'qi' to flow through the body, which is believed to be our principal energy force flowing through us.

It is an important priority to maintain a good balance of chi, and this is why humans indulge in activities such as yoga or meditation. Their meridian network, like an empath's cortex, is also highly sensitive. Think of an empath's energy network as close to how their brain functions, whether it's their chakras or their meridians. The brain of the empath is hypersensitive to stimulators; they are no different in their energy flow.

'Empaths' energy streams are not only susceptible to whatever happens to them directly, but also to the energy of other people. Empaths will also perceive their energy to be unbalanced and require healing because of this. This is why recharging and spending time alone is so necessary for empaths so as to clean their energies somewhat. It is also very important, however, for empaths to know different healing techniques that they can apply to their energy networks, which we will go over in the next section.

THE HEALING ENERGY FOR EMPATHS

Having developed the idea of energy psychiatry, Dr. Orloff believes that energy healing is a very effective addition to other methods of health care, and especially for empaths. Orloff believes that intuition development is key to both healing oneself and healing others, and that it is a method that can be learned and practiced to do so. Anyone should then focus on and develop their intuition, regardless of whether it naturally comes to them or not. You are taking the first step to heal by having a powerful intuition, simply by being able to become more in tune with your energies and thoughts to see how specifically you need to heal.

Even if you believe that you are naturally hypersensitive to subtle energy, either in yourself or in others, because you are not encouraged to use it, this skill may be pushed down or dormant within. When you are able to become more in tune with your energies and feelings, growing your intuition can, in itself, be a step towards healing.

Doing so also helps you to learn how to create hurdles that discourage harmful energy from impacting you as profoundly as it can currently impact you. This is also a calming type in that it allows you to feel a better sense of power. A common fight for empaths is a lack of control, especially over their feelings and the way they respond to the expression of energy and feelings around them. Through meditation, energy healing, and manifestation, being more in touch with your own emotions will allow you to feel a greater sense of control. Working on grounding yourself will help you to have more control of your own energy, so you can exercise limits over what energy you allow to reach your personal space.

A 5-step plan for intuitive energy healing has been created by Dr. Judith Orloff, which is especially helpful for empath. This method is basically somewhat similar to manifestation, as it focuses on the premise that the energy you are sending out is the energy you are going to draw (in this case, intuition is). Noticing your feelings, values, and emotions is the first step in this process. Through meditation or dreaming you should look inward, as many of these values that negatively affect your life can also be unconscious belief structures. Like journaling, which is also a great form of artistic expression, meditation is a great way to take inventory of your inner thoughts and belief systems.

As we've already known, body problems in one of the chakras or meridians can be a sign of blocked energy. Taking inventory of your body is another step in healing your resources. Taking into account how you feel in your whole body, not just in your brain, can be a strong predictor of where you need to concentrate.

Certain physical ailments, for example, may be a symptom of an imbalanced chakra. This can mean a problem with your throat chakra if you feel like your throat is blocked or sore. A good way to note the flow of your energy is to tune in to your physical body. When you do this, you can try to sense the chi and energy movement all over the body. A good way to start healing this is through meditation and yoga, all of which increase the flow of energy and bind you to your source.

Orloff also recommends looking inward and asking for input from the inner self (Mason, 2005). By meditating, praying, communicating with nature, etc. we should listen to our inner self and energy source. We can obtain the guidance we seek from our inner source of energy by doing this regularly and reflecting afterwards, especially with certain questions or manifestations in mind. Lastly, Orloff recommends using dreams as a way to communicate with your inner being and start channeling your energies and healing. One strategy for doing this is to reflect on a question or goal right before you go to bed. Then, right when you wake up, record your dream while it is all fresh in your mind. This will encourage you to contemplate the unconscious responses your brain has given you. By concentrating every night on the same question or purpose, you'll find yourself healing, gaining from the sense of control and continuity.

Although these are just a few steps in a guide to intuitive healing, to tap into your intuition and start healing your energy, there are many processes that you can repeat and practice. You would be able to really look inward by grounding yourself and see if you are internalizing the energies around you. It is important to do this so that you can authentically differentiate the energy that is yours from the energy you have internalized from other people. By doing this, you'll feel much more in charge, especially if you regularly do so. It might seem like a lot of work to constantly look inwards in order to take inventory of your emotions and resources, but once you get the hang of it, it will seem like second nature. Doing so would also greatly help you, helping you to feel more concentrated and in control.

Grounding activities are also quite critical to empath. Empaths will also find themselves tangled up, exhausted, and overstimulated with other people's energies and emotions. To prevent this, it is important to perform various grounding exercises to stay in contact with your inner self and instincts, and not to get caught up in other people's emotions and energies. Breathwork is only one basic grounding technique. Wherever you feel stressed and like you need to get back in touch with your inner energy source, you can practice this practically anywhere.

If you get anxious, you can start by taking a few slow breaths, counting as you inhale for three seconds and as you exhale for three seconds. Repeating this five times will help you get back to the present moment and concentrate on your breath's movements, which will connect you to your inner flow of energy.

Another common grounding approach focuses on the senses, which are hypersensitive to empath. Focusing on every sense as a way of grounding yourself will allow you to be very much in tune with your inner energies and the way you are linked to the present moment. You need to pay attention to your surroundings with this technique, called the 5-4-3-2-1 technique. First, take some deep breaths and then take in the surroundings, beginning by recognizing five objects you can see. Then recognize four things that you can touch and feel, three sounds that you can hear, two things that you can smell, and one that you can taste. A perfect way to hold yourself in the present moment and stop being too distracted by the energy you are taking in is to concentrate on these various feelings as they apply to your environment.

CHAPTER 7:

SELF-CARE FOR EMPATHS

Self-care is one of the most significant moves you will take in healing as an empath. In order to provide about other people, empaths often find themselves neglecting their own needs. Empaths are also people who care about other people, support them, and heal them, but this can make them neglect to healing and care about themselves. In reality, in order to adequately care for others, it is extremely necessary to prioritize their own health. We find ourselves less successful at our work and having difficulty in our relationships when we neglect our own self-care.

It can be difficult not to be overwhelmed by the negative energy that you are trying to heal, particularly as an empath, being in a role where your primary task is to healing or care for others. In addition, these caregivers very frequently spend so much time with other individuals that they can begin to forget where their feelings end and where the feelings of other people begin. You are not yourself, if you ignore your own self-care for too long. We will go over the importance of self-care for empaths in this chapter, and the techniques that you can do regularly to protect your resources. Both empaths are, to a degree, narrators with high intensity. The word "high-intensity relator," coined by Howard Brockman, a social worker, and author, refers to any entity who, in an interpersonal sense, takes on the role of a caregiver.

As a career, these individuals take on healing and caring for others. Even if you are not expected to do this by your occupation, you are likely to take on this role in many of your interpersonal relationships as an empath. Although this position is what you are gravitating towards and what ultimately delivers fulfillment to you, it can be stressful and overwhelming. In addition, when you ignore your own well-being, you will find yourself less successful in these positions. Just as being too selfish can have a negative influence on your lifestyle, you can find that being too centered on other people will potentially also have negative effects on you.

Although this may sound contradictory, since we can all aspire to be less narcissistic, the way you and others view yourself may also alter a lack of self-awareness. Spending time caring for yourself and healing your own energies will encourage you to look inward and see if, by working outward, you can be more successful. Self-care is an important priority for any human being, but especially for empaths. They will find themselves feeling lost, frustrated, and out of control of their feelings if empaths do not prioritize self-care. Have you ever started to cry for no reason, or felt really on-edge even though you didn't have anything unique going on that made you feel stressed? There are normal things that can happen when empaths get anxious and overwhelmed. This is why self-care needs to be prioritized in order to avoid burnout. While at first, it will seem like a lot of effort and energy, you can see that this path of your energy is extremely worth it, especially in the long run.

In addition, doing this kind of job will make you vulnerable to emotional contagion. If after you care about others, you don't know how to care for yourself as an empath, you can find yourself internalizing and experiencing the negative trauma of others too profoundly. Part of being a caregiver or a healer means to some degree removing yourself from the problem you are trying to work on, so that you can support someone else effectively. Although the ability to empathize is crucial to helping another person, since this can have detrimental consequences, you do not want to find yourself getting caught up in the discomfort they can experience. To stop falling into a rut because of the internalization of others' feelings, first, you need to take care of yourself.

Where things may also get tough on empath is when you find yourself unintentionally internalizing others' feelings. This is why time alone is so vital to empath. Even if you are taking steps to prioritize your own self-care, but still constantly find yourself surrounded by other people, even if you are not technically on the clock and functioning as a caregiver, you might still be internalizing their resources. As we've already learned, being an empath is a blessing and gives you many spiritual and interpersonal skills, as well as many life skills. This is not a bad thing. It only means, however, that you need to make sure that you prioritize your self-care and in-kind recharging.

Brockman also addresses the word 'compassion exhaustion,' referring to the symptoms that empath and/or caregivers can suffer too much while internalizing the suffering and/or trauma of others. Also, it is critical that you regularly prioritize self-care. If you're just regularly engaging in things that can help you sporadically relax and deal with stress, you won't get into a healthy routine, and you'll probably find yourself dealing with a lot of the same issues you've helped others function through.

You may be thinking to yourself that all of this sounds very self-explanatory and straightforward after reading through this section. If you feel down, shouldn't you do the things that make you feel better? And it should seem like a simple instinct. But this is obviously not as simple as it sounds for empaths in particular.

Empaths spend so much time concentrating their energies and attention on other people that they just don't even think about turning these resources into themselves for healing and caregiving. Empaths might also hope to find this satisfaction in other people, instead opting to pursue the feelings of self-care in their relationship with others, rather than in their relationship with themselves.

Empaths are often very used to placing the wishes and concerns of others above their own. They also find themselves being forced to the side because of this. We prefer to dismiss self-care as trivial or insignificant in our busy lives, when it's really one of the most important things we can do. Part of this is also because we see compassion for others and compassion for ourselves as entirely separate mechanisms, whereas they are very similar fundamentally. A significant part of this is self-awareness. While you growing assume that you are self-aware because you are focused on others as an empath, this is not actually the case. Self-awareness can also be a chance to be empathic, as deciding the feelings and energies are your own and which are those of other people can often be challenging. Part of self-care is to note, and then act intuitively on, which of these emotions are yours. But you must know your instincts in order to use your instincts. And this comes from an understanding of oneself, which is basically self-care.

Self-compassion is also linked to another type of self-care that researchers have researched and come to conclusions about, which is basically at the heart of self-care. Self-compassion is the answer you need to fully grasp your intuition and what it is. While the self-care that appears "pleasant," such as yoga or acupuncture, or journaling, is necessary and extremely helpful, the more complicated types of self-care are also important to practice. This could involve having difficult talks with yourself about what habits you should alter and what does not serve you any longer. But this can also involve having these hard discussions in your life with the people.

Even if it isn't easy, self-care can mean cutting out toxic people, such as energy vampires, from your life. If anyone takes advantage of your empathic tendencies, in order to have more resources to concentrate on the relationships that are actually supporting you, you will need to prioritize yourself and cut them out of your life. Although this is challenging, there are many benefits to the practice of self-compassion. In reality, research also shows that showing compassion for yourself can work to minimize various psychological problems and help you manage stress better.

If all this still sounds like a foreign language to you, it's all right; we're going to go through a lot of different self-care strategies that, in the next segment, you can start incorporating into your routine. But if you ever wonder how you can even make self-care a big part of your routine, then that's all right too. You might say, "But I barely have time for food. How can I find the time to meditate every day, and do yoga?" But it all comes down to preferences to address this question. First, you need to start putting yourself first and genuinely believe that the most important thing is self-care. If you really internalize and believe this, you will find all your energies gravitating to your self-care, and it won't be hard to make time to put yourself first. Know, you need to start showing the same kindness to yourself as you display to other people. When you begin to love yourself more, you'll find yourself with greater love to give to others.

TECHNIQUES FOR SELF-CARE

There are countless ways to take care of yourself, your body, mind and spirit, and whatever means you want to engage regularly are up to you. There are, however, some types of self-care that are especially beneficial for the empath in particular, and some that doctors and therapists also prescribe. Whatever kinds of self-care you want to do to de-stress and refresh, make sure you set up a strong routine and ensure that you consistently prioritize yourself. Consistency is crucial here—there is not one "true" way to care for yourself, but if you don't make it a priority to be consistent, you won't be pleased with the results.

Spending time alone is an especially powerful technique for empath, as we have already established several times in this book, as they often get distracted and over-stimulated while spending too much time with others. Therefore, performing some task in isolation is a perfect way for empaths to take care of themselves, by using their instincts and getting back in touch with their own unique needs. Specifically, Dr. Orloff recommends not just spending time alone but also blocking out any potential stimulators that are hypersensitive to the senses. This involves turning off your television, switching off any bright lights, and getting away from any location where other people surround you.

It is also a good idea to surround yourself with nature, since empaths are also very energized by nature and find their energies being cleansed by nature. Empaths are also recharged around water, so going to a water body can be a great way of self-care as well. Even though empaths crave human interaction, you may find it a good idea to shut the interaction off for a little while when you prioritize your alone time. You will discover that it will encourage you to really spend time with your thoughts to silence your phone and go for a walk alone. This, in turn, will help you discern your true source of energy, and without distracting energy from others, you can use your instincts to get in contact with your thoughts and feelings. It will also make your decisions more effective, as you will concentrate on your values, thoughts, and what you want, rather than the emotions of other people around you.

Another type of self-care is setting limits for empaths that can be integrated into your everyday life. For anyone, this is an essential life skill, not just empath, but it is incredibly necessary to preserve your resources from emotional contagion and "energy vampires." This is an essential life skill. It will help you to prioritize and protect your personal well-being from anyone who might be taking advantage of you by setting limits on when and how you interact. When you give too much to others and encourage them to stress you too much, even though you are a helper at heart, this can adversely affect any aspect of your life. You can find yourself so burdened, at its most extreme, that you struggle emotionally, psychologically, and even physically. And you will not be a productive caregiver or healer to others while you are suffering. Think of how you can quickly recognize that someone close to you has something wrong—they can also recognize this in you.

For this purpose, making yourself, your health, and your instincts, your top priorities is extremely important. If this involves distancing yourself for a time and setting limits, then these acts must be done to potentially benefit everyone. It might not seem like setting boundaries is a form of self-care given that it also includes your relationships with others. Since empaths are so relationship-focused, however, self-care undoubtedly requires the development of healthy boundaries and behaviors within your relationships. By setting clear intentions on what you feel is necessary to prioritize, you can start doing this gradually. You will get into the habit of doing this in your relationships until you start setting limits, and you will be able to see the advantages.

Something you certainly have learned time and time again is one of the most significant factors in your well-being: having enough sleep. Sleep is the manner in which we really "recharge." Even if you follow all the other advice in this book, if you don't get enough sleep, you won't be well balanced and safe. That's science—sleep can help you remain physically, mentally, and spiritually healthiest. A lack of sleep can also cause you to consume more negative energy, according to Orloff. When you are deprived of much-needed rest, have you ever found yourself much more on-edge and vulnerable to consuming negative energy? It is a known fact that when we don't get enough sleep, we don't do as well as we should, in anything.

In addition, sleep can bring many benefits as it relates to dreaming and healing energy. The more one sleeps, the more one dreams. In the most common sense, this heals your energy, spirit, and physical wellbeing, which is self-care. If you're feeling out of sorts and stressed out, you can also listen to several directed sleep meditations while you close your eyes, which will help your brain unconsciously heal your energy when you're sleeping. Note, 7-8 hours of sleep a night is essential for the average adult. This type of self-care is not a privilege, but a requirement (as with all forms of self-care). If you don't sleep enough, you don't do one of the most essential things you can do to safeguard your overall health.

Another excellent approach for self-care is journaling, especially for empaths. Journalizing is an incredible and therapeutic way of sharing the thoughts and imagination. It will also encourage you to really tap into your instincts, as you are validating and recognizing where your thoughts and energies lie by writing down anything and everything that comes to mind. Journalizing is also an important manifestation technique. This will help you imagine what you desire, and how you will feel when you have attracted this thing by writing down what you expect to manifest. It also validates what you are seeking to manifest, and when you strive to attract that feeling, it solidifies the connection to the world. Journaling is a perfect way to work through and recognize any feelings you might be uncertain about, especially for empaths.

Another excellent strategy of self-care to maximize the flow of your positive energies is showing gratitude. With journaling or meditation, this can be achieved and is necessary for manifestation. You may find that you can start looking at your situation in a more optimistic light by reflecting on everything in your life that you are thankful for, and whatever might be causing you stress will no longer seem quite as bad. You may boost an attitude that could have turned pessimistic due to energy vampires or emotional contagion by showing gratitude.

Therapy is another kind of self-care that may directly help empaths or other extremely sensitive individuals. Since empaths are usually the "therapists" in their relationships, being the ones other people go to for guidance and problem-solving, a lot of their own problems and trauma can be swept under the rug. It can, therefore be immensely helpful to see a therapist, even if it only provides you with someone to speak to. Therapists are also helpful in providing us with support to work with any mental illnesses we can suffer from. Going to therapy is a perfect way to unpack some pent-up emotional trauma so that the tension and negative feelings you might be internalizing from the people around you will avoid weighing you down. Therapy is known to help your interpersonal relationships and problem-solving abilities, so if you still struggle to bear the weight that empaths sometimes hold, it might be important for you to reach out to a therapist.

In addition, as an empath, you can be vulnerable to attracting vampires of energy who repeatedly speak your ear off and unload their baggage onto you. You will lighten this charge a little bit by going to the counseling, freeing up space to focus on your own intuitive energies. You will also find that focusing on your intuitive talents becomes simpler for you, as you have more resources to concentrate on the things that matter to you. You can find that a lot of doors open up for you when you start unpacking your inner emotions.

In the context of practicing spirituality, you should also integrate self-care into your routine, to support both your body and mind. Self-care means checking in and seeing where you can enhance your physical well-being. Exercise is a perfect way to clear your mind and alleviate tension, since it not only helps your body, but also activates endorphins, increases your vitality, and cleanses it. Another type of self-care is calming your chakras, which you can physically, spiritually, and emotionally benefit from.

You can also embed a lot of these strategies into your sleep. You will clear up your energy as you sleep, wake up refreshed and energized in the morning by listening to various guided sleep meditations as you doze off. Of course, you should concentrate on the various spiritual activities that work for you. You can notice, for example, that you hate meditation, but you love to do yoga. Whatever habits you think encourage your well-being in the best way possible, make sure to do them as much as you can and really create a routine. Just how to work out once a month simply won't be as productive as creating a fitness routine a few days a week on a daily basis, so you have to do the same for your spirituality to really see the benefits.

Although these are actually only a few self-care strategies for empaths, there are a multitude of other ways you may take some time to refresh yourself periodically. Whatever works for you, inside and without your spirit and body, you will find that it enhances the flow of your energy. We will concentrate on how you should apply the concept of self-care directly to various sources of energy and healing in these next pages.

Healing is a major part of the technique of self-care. Without prioritizing ourselves, we can't heal our resources, and this can mean feeling like you put certain parts of your life on hold. But note, you'll see that all of your relationships will end up winning in return when you put yourself first. You are also prioritizing your relationships with other people by prioritizing yourself, and you are learning how to give your best self.

CHAPTER 8:

HOW TO RE-CHANNEL YOUR EMPATH ENERGY

Now that we've addressed the importance of giving priority to self-care, you might have agreed that you're ready to start concentrating your attention on your own personal well-being. But you may also think to yourself that this is likely to be much easier said than done, and that is a fair point. It's not an easy feat to re-channel energy to yourself that you've been guiding into other people for your whole life. Energy healing is a process, not something that comes easily, and learning how to really tap into our energy sources and guide it into our own personal well-being requires a lot of work and practice.

The empath appears to ignore itself, instead focusing all of its attention on others. But you can ultimately tap into a source of true abundance by focusing some of your energies on healing yourself. You'll find that you have an abundance of love and joy to give out, rather than running yourself thin as empaths appear to do. Simply accessing and redirecting this energy stream is the secret to accessing this energy and using your intuitive gifts, which we will learn how to do in the next chapters.

But first, let's talk a little more about what healing energy really is. We have already discussed meridians and chakras and how they dictate the energy flow, and we have decided what chi is. But let's now describe how some of the mechanisms behind actually repairing the energy flow of the body function. As an alternative psychiatric healing type, one common holistic type of energy healing is Reiki energy healing. A therapeutic therapy that works to heal the mind, body, and spirit is Reiki energy healing. A lot of the ways in which our energy flows across our body, as we have learned, depend not only on the mind but also on the physical being. Reiki healing, which a Japanese man discovered, focuses on this connection. The healing type focuses on blocked or turned negative energy flows in the body, and heals them, rendering them constructive.

This technique, as an empath, can be especially helpful because it helps release internalized negative energy. All too often, empaths feel they have unconsciously internalized other people's harmful energy. Although non-empaths may be more selective with the energy that reaches their bodies, simply because they are less prone to stimulants, empaths internalize the feelings and energies of other people at a much higher level. Reiki healing acts primarily to elevate the vibrations surrounding the points of harmful energy in the body, helping an empath expel all of those feelings that have been internalized unconsciously.

By relaxation, Reiki also helps to relieve tension and feelings of pain, eventually improving the vibrations throughout the body. It also helps to remove any energy blockages in the body, allowing energy to circulate more easily inside and outside. This applies the body to holistic therapy and energy balance. Reiki healing, while not once considered a real medical procedure, has now been researched widely and is even being provided at some hospitals. You will possibly locate a nearby practitioner near you if you are trying to obtain Reiki healing, because it is a medical as well as holistic activity.

Pranic healing is another popular and widely used method of energy healing. In that it does not take a hands-on approach to heal the energy flows of the body, this method of energy healing varies from Reiki healing. Pranic healing, instead, retains the idea that the body will heal itself by various methods depending on whatever health condition you suffer from. Pranic healing holds the belief system that our energy source, called Prana, flows inside and outside the body, and that our body can repair any possible blockages. This method of healing focuses on various areas of the energy field of the body that may be impacted by a blockage. For example, if you were to go in to see a pranic healer with a problem involving your lower back or the base of your spine, the healer will probably concentrate on your root chakra and try to restore the energy that flows in this energy field region.

Both forms of energy healing, though they have different techniques, are widely popularized. There are also countless other methods of energy healing, and it will take self-awareness and rely on your personal interests to choose the right one for you. There are also ways, however, in which you can work to balance your own flows of energy, which we will discuss in the following sections.

WHY AND HOW SHOULD WE LEARN TO REDIRECT ENERGY?

Although we've talked about some common forms of professional energy healing, there are also ways you can work to redirect the negative energy in your own body. In this method, the first step includes consciously and intuitively recognizing when you internalize negative energy around you. You possibly already have a good intuition as an empath. However, when an emotion is naturally yours, and when it is someone else's, it can often be hard to say. Therefore, to decide how to heal your own powers, you need to take some time alone to meditate on your thoughts, emotions, and intentions. Staying conscious and aware of how your energy affects your mood and your life is crucial. Since empaths are so prone without even realizing it to internalize energy around them, staying conscious and self-aware is extra essential. That's why journaling and meditation are excellent resources to keep in contact with your particular area of energy and with the processes taking place in your mind and body. These acts allow you to observe your ideas and the energy that flows through you.

To start cleaning up your energy and generally freeing up any blockages without concentrating on any particular points, you must first sit down with your thoughts and note them. To do this, meditating or spending time alone in nature will benefit you. Your thoughts can reflect the flow of energy in your body, because the most concentrated thoughts are the ones you offer the most energy. This, in essence, absorbs more of anything you concentrate on, as the Law of Attraction teaches us that the thoughts you offer the most power to become the ones you pull into your life.

Your personal belief systems must also be tested. What are you working on, and what are you no longer serving at this time? Noticing just what the energy is being directed to can help you learn how to heal it. You will need to concentrate on being aware and alert—this can sometimes be challenging for empaths, since their first impulse is to concentrate all of their energy on others' emotions. With practice, however, you will build focus rather than outer stimulants to your inner movement. It is precisely a lack of conscious awareness that can aggravate an energy imbalance, so the first step to healing is awareness.

If you still have problems determining where you can try to channel the energy in your life, try to think about various aspects of it. You may feel like you've never had a day off work, and you're working overtime constantly, but you somehow seem broken. In this scenario, your energy could be blocked because it has to do with abundance in your life. You may also use the Law of Attraction and techniques of manifestation to increase the healing of your energy. But that is what you pull into your life by dwelling on the lack of resources you have. It is necessary to express gratitude and start framing things from a beneficial light in order to start healing the way your energy flows. Concentrate on the appreciation you have for your work and the ability to raise money instead of dwelling on the feeling of losing money. You will find that the negative energy surrounding this part of your life is healed by this. You may extend this to various spheres of your life, including relationships. It is also important that you explore, as an empath, the way energy flows through your various interpersonal relationships. Do you have any relationships that you believe to be the only one that brings energy into that relationship, but you sometimes end up with negative feelings about it? This could be a sign that you need to re-examine who and what deserves your time and energy.

It is important to always keep an eye on what we put our resources into. If we find, however, that this does not benefit us, we should begin learning to redirect where our energy is being channeled. This can be hard to understand as an empath, because the first impulse of an empath is to focus all of their energies on understanding and supporting others. This, though, is counterintuitive to your own recovery, and that can potentially make you the kind of negative person you're trying to stop.

It is a perfect method of self-care to distance yourself from this toxic energy, and you can see the positive results. You may also take several steps to protect your own resources from any environmental factors. This will allow you to track any trends that you have observed so as not to impede your personal development.

HOW TO HEAL AND PREVENT ENERGY BLOCKAGES

Now that we have discussed some energy blockage clearing strategies, let's backtrack and explore how "blocked" our energy can even become. Some signs of energy blockage might be so widespread to you that you don't even know how very critical they are. One common sign of blocking the flow of energy is realizing that the thoughts are trapped. This is also a common sign of an anxiety disorder, and empaths will struggle with this frequently. Having thoughts that are stuck or focused on one thing, and finding yourself incapable of thinking about something else or taking your mind off the topic, may imply a blockage in this area of your life.

Why can't you resist gravitating into that one area of your life? It's important to find out what it's that will help you get "unstuck," even if you're not yet there. You can recreate the feeling of it until you can imagine what it is that will take your mind off this fixed thinking. For example, maybe you're concerned about a test you've just taken, and can't seem to stop thinking about it, even though you've already turned it in. You know if you got a good grade on it, you can stop thinking about the exam. So, to get "unstuck" from this needless energy waste, imagine the feeling you might have when you find out that on this exam, you got a good score. Then internalize this feeling and substitute the nervous feeling about the exam with the optimistic feeling.

You should concentrate on the flow of energy in each particular chakra as well. If you know that you could be vulnerable to energy blocks in your heart chakra as an empath, then incorporating ways to prioritize self-care that will directly impact your heart chakra will be a smart idea. In addition, as we'll discuss in the next chapter, you may still feel the effects of past trauma that has built up and never been completely resolved. If you do not completely prioritize healing and clear this trapped energy, it will only intensify the positions where you encounter blockages and continue to affect your life in various ways. In other aspects of your life, this can also impair the flow of positive energy.

It might also be difficult for you to discern where you have blocked energy, since you are so prone to internalizing other people's energy. While this can also generate obstacles, these blockages are not usually the same as the energetic and emotional blockages arising from pent-up and unhealed trauma. To start prioritizing your healing process, it is important that you explore the areas of your life in which you are not absolutely happy. You find yourself continually repeating the same bad habits, even though you try to break them consciously? In the forms of procrastination, these bad habits will manifest, deliberately sabotaging relationships, and even over-eating.

A good way to start healing your blocked energy is by making a list of all the places of your life that don't seem to have healthy, free-flowing energy. You can also find like you should get near to new ideas at times—why do you think this is so? By finding places where you have been most affected by pent-up emotional distress, you will start healing effectively. Some of these blockages can also influence your physical health and well-being, as we have discovered that in different areas of the body, different chakras are concentrated.

Crystal healing is a helpful way to focus on avoiding energy blockages and healing any aspects you think may be blocked. This is another common type of alternative medicine, as different crystals are believed to have various effects on our energy flows. It is claimed that crystals facilitate the flow of energy in our body and can help rid the body of any negative pent-up energy. Different crystals have different functions and can be used to help avoid energy blockages in different ways. For example, you may want to meditate with a rose quartz stone or hold it by your bed while you sleep if you strive to enhance the flow of love in your life and sometimes find you have trouble in relationships. If, as can sometimes happen to empaths, you want to stop harmful energy from entering your energy field, you can find it beneficial to start meditating with and holding citrine. You will be able to protect your healthy, constructive energies from external threats to your inner peace with this stone.

There are also several empathic strategies, in particular, to avoid the entry of harmful and destructive energies into their minds and bodies. Boundary-setting is one perfect way to do this. In the nature of empaths, boundary-setting is always not, as they instinctively seek closeness with others and enjoy becoming healers and/or caregivers. To protect your own energy, however, doing this is extremely necessary. Think of it as forming a protective shield around your energy field—you don't want to get contaminants that can easily get in and contaminate anything around them. By looking at where you can start building healthy boundaries in your relationships, you can find that you are expressing much more positive energy, which is what you will gain in return. This probably goes without saying too, but resources can be easily preserved by taking on more self-care. When you become more in tune with your feelings, emotions, and instincts, permeating your spirit becomes harder for the negative energy.

Another important way to preserve your energy flows is by training yourself to note energy without responding to it initially. In meditation, this can also be practiced, when you note a thought and then simply let it go without listening or reacting to it. Often your first impulse will be to respond to stimuli, always trying to support people when you feel you will. It is necessary, however, to first take note of how you are impacted by energy and emotions. It is important to keep track of what energy is circulating around you and how you internalize it to choose how you can react best when you choose to do so. Since empaths can often think with their hearts and not with their brains, they can often act on feelings impulsively. However, you can feel much more in control of your own energy patterns by keeping track and really understanding the rhythm of your emotions and energy, and what is triggering these reactions in you.

Another way you can stop energy blockages is by changing your attitude as it relates to other individuals. Obviously, as an empath, you want to support others. But are you ever feeling like trying to improve them or helping them to solve problems in vain?

You can have to contend with the fact that some people are just the way they are. An overinvestment in other individuals might lead to less satisfaction for both, as you could feel as if no progress is being made, and they could feel like you are attempting to improve them unfairly. Letting go of other people's desires is a perfect way to start redirecting the energies into your own instincts and health. It's also an unproductive way of trying to get leverage. While empaths frequently attempt to gain control of their lives and circumstances, it is never beneficial for anyone to try to manipulate other people's thoughts, emotions, and behaviors. Instead, monitor the ways in which you respond to their feelings and internalize them. By focusing inwards, you can also achieve this sense of control over your resources. Although you can not control the fact that you are inherently an empath, you can control the ways you react to the energies and emotions of other people. You will find the power that you seek by enhancing your own sense of intuition.

And note, without self-care, there is no energy healing. The two go hand-in-hand, and you have to start prioritizing self-care if you want to begin to change the way your energy flows and redirect what your attention goes to. Through doing so, you'll be able to uncover your unconscious thoughts and feelings that could surprise you. At first, this may also be daunting, but it will ultimately be incredibly worth it, because, in every aspect of your life, you will reap the benefits.

CHAPTER 9:

THE GIFT OF HEALING AS AN EMPATH

While we have already explored several different ways of energy healing, it is important to wrap up this guide by understanding the value of cherishing and cultivating your intuitive gifts by tapping into your intuition. As we have already known, because of a lack of motivation in our society, many empaths feel that their innate intuitive talents have been silenced or made to lie dormant. This, coupled with the potential trauma that you may face from the continuous internalization of the negative energy and emotions of other people, may lead to feelings of helplessness or hopelessness. Yet, healing is possible. The first step in curing these gifts is to continue to read this book and consciously pay more attention to your inner source of energy and intuition. You are taking a significant first step towards prioritizing your own well-being and putting yourself first by noting that you can maximize the energy flows in your life. Now, let's talk about some common traumas that you may find yourself particularly vulnerable to as an empath.

Dr. Orloff says one of the first steps toward recovery is to recognize what kind of empath you think you are. Are you more of a mental, or physical empath? Orloff describes physical empath as someone who is more in touch with others' physical emotions, and that's how they interact with the energy sources of others. The "super empaths" we discussed earlier in this book, for example, would classify as physical empaths. Usually, actual empaths are capable of actively internalizing others' emotions. For example, if a friend suffers from a physical ailment, an empath may be able to feel some of this pain in their own body internally. This also suggests, though, that emotional empath will also pick up on that well-being when someone feels physically well.

In comparison, an emotional empath senses other people's feelings just as intensely as the primary sensation. This tends to be more prominent in empath. For example, many people can feel better about their own lives, but they can find themselves internalizing these negative emotions as though they were their own though they spend time around someone who radiates negative emotions. This is why learning how to protect your own energy is extremely necessary, so you are at less risk of experiencing the detrimental effects of the pain and feelings of other people. Emotional feelings also fail to distinguish the overlap between their emotions and the emotions of other people. But this doesn't mean you have to cut other people out of your life as an empath, just because they are sad. Instead, it means you can just start focusing on preserving your own energy, so you can maintain a strong relationship without actually allowing your energy field to be permeated by their negativity.

One strong way to start healing your energy from any invading forces is not just to set limits, but actually to use the Law of Attraction as well as visualization to really keep your energy secure from those around you. It is important to look inwards first and really explore where your feelings and thoughts begin and where other people's emotions end. In reality, you can then imagine yourself setting up a boundary around your energy and severing energetic relations with others' energy fields in a sense. You can also show empath by manifesting this, without experiencing precisely what other people feel to the same extent.

To do this, a simple exercise is to take deep breaths first, relax yourself, and concentrate on the flow of your breath. Think of this as meditation, as you strive to bring yourself into the relaxed, centered headspace. Then you can start imagining yourself building a defensive forcefield around you to keep your energy protected from external forces. In order to stop their energy from influencing you as much as it does, you can also imagine yourself cutting energetic links with another person. You can imagine that your energies are connected by a rope and that this rope is cut with scissors. In helping you to ground yourself and preserve your energetic dignity, these visualization exercises can be very beneficial.

There are many ways you can unlearn harmful habits that may have developed as a result of trauma, as well as build new strategies for coping and healing to help you move forward. But the first step to do this is to unpack what has caused you trauma so you can figure out how to better recover. A particular process would be to heal trauma due to fear of becoming particular due to trauma from an abusive relationship. By knowing where the trauma comes from and how it currently affects the energy flows, you will begin to see where those blocks of energy come from and how you can repair them. Doing this would be an excellent first step as an empath on your journey to recovery. You can begin by meditating and journaling. Doing a grounding meditation is a great way to get in touch with your inner thoughts and feelings, particularly those you might not recognize on the surface. By paying attention to how you feel and how your energy tends to flow through various sectors of your life, you can gain a lot of insight into what you can focus on and what does not help you any longer.

In addition, empaths may begin to internalize trauma from dysfunctional relationships. Empaths are simply magnets for vampires of energy trying to take advantage of them. This can have a great effect on their well-being, as the trauma associated with the relationship can show itself in other relationships as difficulties. In our relationships, however, there are ways to heal. It is not only possible to ground yourself and start healing yourself from inside, but it is also possible to have discussions with people close to you about the trauma that you might be going through to recover together.

You should start analyzing your relationships to see how the energy in each one of them flows. If you have any relationships with energy vampires at the present moment, that's the first place to look is. One symptom of pent-up trauma is that you might find yourself continuing the pattern of constantly beginning relationships with energy vampires, subconsciously enabling them to permeate and take advantage of your energy sector. The first step to healing in this respect, as we've learned, is through self-reflection. The best way for you to begin to recover would eventually be self-reflection and the practice of your empathic intuitive gifts.

THE COMMON TRAUMAS THAT EMPATHS EXPERIENCE

There are many traumatic events that empath is particularly vulnerable to. You are however, well placed on the road to recovery through knowing and recognizing what these kinds of trauma can be. Having a list of anything you feel may be an issue with your energy is vital. Do you find that in social situations you get especially nervous and have a hunch that you might be susceptible to social anxiety?

Take account thereof. Do you ever find that you internalize feelings of sadness when you're around someone sad, which can exacerbate your own emotions? Also, take care of that. Empaths are also very vulnerable to social anxiety due to their susceptibility to stimuli. They can pick up on the most subtle energies, noting items that might not be heard by others. Because of this, the empath in social settings can get very easily stressed and overwhelmed, particularly as children, when they only learn to use their instincts and probably don't understand their gifts (Orloff, 2018). This is one common trauma facing empath, as it can be daunting and stimulating to the point of avoidance to be in large numbers of people and in crowds.

Fear of rejection is another common empathic trauma (Orloff, 2018). Ultimately, empaths are people who crave an intimate bond with others. This can affect them far more profoundly and impactfully than non-empaths when they feel as though they are being rejected. Even if it's a non-personal rejection, such as a missed job opportunity, the empath will also feel the consequences of rejection to the deepest degree. This may be another case of an empath being accused of being "too sensitive," or appearing to take something beyond expectations. However, the explanation for this is simply that empaths profoundly crave emotional interaction, and rejection feels like a rejection of that.

The impression that they are not really themselves, or that they are living out of fear of not being accepted, is another particular type of trauma that empaths can be influenced by beyond childhood. This can come through several years of learning to inhibit their empathic ability, which can manifest in adulthood as being unable to fully be yourself or as emotionally shutting yourself off. It is important to get back into contact with your instincts and energy source in order to move beyond this, to start tapping back into your natural gifts and emotions. To do this, there are many healing methods that can be performed.

Another cause of empathic trauma may be their relationships with people who steal their life from them, or life vampires. These individuals can cause an empath to feel taken advantage of, drained, and generally cause them to consume much negative energy. That can be a kind of abusive relationship as well. Emotionally abusive relationships can provide a source of unhealed empathic trauma, creating difficulty for them to develop new connections and thrive in future relationships. This is another field in which focusing on redirecting and healing your energy flows as they relate to other individuals is significant.

Many empaths will also become empath as a result of violence they as children may have faced. This can be an exceedingly frustrating thing that they would then work on in adulthood. For example, certain empaths are hypersensitive even to other people's smallest shifts, which is basically how they were eventually able to say whether they were in danger. While this sensing threat ability is an advantage to being empathic, being abused may be the unfortunate reason behind learning this ability. Thus, this trauma will carry on into their later lives, causing empaths to find themselves very on-edge and hypersensitive to something they feel could be a threat to them, even though it is not. This can be a kind of "side effect" of being an empath and explains a lot of why other people can find empaths more guarded or closed-off, simply because they are so sensitive to potential threats. Empaths may also, for this purpose, grow what is known as paranoia. It can be written off as paranoia, even though they are always correct about their instincts, since they are the first to feel a person or situation's real and subtle energy. This may also lead them to have their natural instincts quite blocked, not wanting to trust it for fear of becoming paranoid, which can manifest as unhealed trauma in adulthood.

The propensity to consume all the emotions around them is another common trauma that empathizes experience, due to a lack of grounding and healing. This can make them feel taken for granted, or like they let people walk all over them. This can strengthen a feeling of helplessness later in life when they repeatedly let toxic people take them for granted and drain them of energy, especially earlier in life. Empaths will also find that, simply because of the behaviors they developed as children, they have difficulty standing up for themselves or saying no to people. However, you can preserve your own energy enough by focusing on setting limits and grounding yourself to where you can know what should and should not be accessing your energy field.

Having empathic gifts, as we have already mentioned, can also be a pathway to self-destructive habits, such as getting into unhealthy relationships and addiction continuously. Empaths also learn that they are trying to "numb the suffering" that comes with being an empath. This can result in harmful actions, since they can not cope with the emotions of being continually over-stimulated. For an empath, this is why self-care is so critical. It's important that they find ways by which they channel and convey their own and other feelings, so that they don't feel frustrated and disturbed by the weight they bear.

TECHNIQUES FOR EMPATHS HEALING

While there are quite a few common habits that can block an empathic force, there are a variety of methods and techniques that can be used to heal the force. A better technique is certainly simpler than it sounds—to note and take stock of your thoughts and feelings when you feel them. This is said so much easier than done, when no one wants to think consciously about every thought they have, contemplating why and how they feel every emotion that crosses their mind. You may, therefore, deliberately integrate these acts into your routine of self-care. Try to take yourself some time to meditate and to focus on your feelings. Journalizing with the intention of differentiating your feelings from other people's feelings is also a brilliant idea. A perfect way to get a sense of control and equilibrium back into your body is to put your emotions in perspective and analyze what it is that makes you feel the way you do. This insight would encourage you to stay empathic, but while you are putting conscious awareness into how they affect your mind, you probably won't be as emotionally affected by the emotions of others.

Orloff recommends repeating the mantra "return to sender" as another technique for healing energy triggered by the trauma of internalizing the feelings of others. When repeating this phrase, it's also important to concentrate on your breath flow, slowly inhale and exhale as you repeat the mantra either aloud or in your mind. This mantra helps to expel any harmful energy from those around you that you've internalized. Repeating this mantra confidently, helps you to guide the energy out of your body. This is a perfect strategy to do when you've been around a big group of people, or just feel a little "off." By guiding this toxic energy out of your mind and body, you'll be better able to concentrate on the energy that comes from you.

Increasing your physical distance is another way of reducing the inflow of toxic and traumatic energy, particularly for a physical empath. If you are in a busy environment and feel out of control of the toxic energies you internalize, you should move away physically and take some time to recharge your battery. In group settings and crowded places, it is important for you to normalize this, especially if you have trauma associated with being in large groups. Many empaths may notice that they explicitly have trauma related to spending too much time with large groups as a child. By reducing physical interaction with other people, another way that you can increase your physical distance is. Since energy is often transmitted through physical touch, you can make the choice to reduce physical contact with other people, particularly those you are not as close to, if you feel like you need to heal your energy and protect your body from internalizing too much toxic external energy.

On an emotional level, you too, can increase your gap. Healing pent-up trauma can also be done by establishing boundaries and limitations on interpersonal contact, as we've already developed. Determining that you need and/or want space from other people is perfectly true. It is completely valid to take some time to remove yourself so that you can recover and isolate your energy from theirs if one of your friends is burdening you with energy that reminds you of a past traumatic event.

Allowing yourself solitary time to regroup and really concentrate on healing is also necessary. Even if you feel as if you are actively prioritizing your self-care, committing to healing is important in reality. This can mean unlearning codependency patterns from the past. Empaths, for example, often find themselves being codependent in their relationships, which may, in turn, lead to more closeness issues. If you're somebody that doesn't know how to be alone comfortably and spend time with yourself, that's possibly the product of the past trauma that you've formed through various empathic features. For just a small amount of time, you can start by sitting alone with your thoughts. A perfect way to refresh and restore your soul from the effects of trauma is also to spend time in nature.

Care to pursue visualization, as well. You may practice various methods of grounding that will help you concentrate your attention on grounding yourself and being in contact with your own attention. It is not a straightforward feat to unlearn trauma. It's hard and can take a lot of time and energy to actively concentrate on unlearning trauma, but working through any energetic barriers you may experience is worth it.

CHAPTER 10:

HOW TO EMBRACE YOUR GIFT

Being an empath is physically and emotionally draining, as you have heard, which can lead you to feel as though you don't have a gift but a responsibility. Feeling this responsibility represents the first step towards acknowledging your gift. You will need to learn how to look after yourself now so that without feeling drained, you can enjoy your gift. This is an incredibly important method, and the best strategies for successful coping mechanisms can be learned with time and effort. If you learn how to cope with and act as empath, you can make use of your gift to change yourself and world.

You must go to great lengths to remove the harmful energies that you might attract, because of the intense feelings of intense emotions and tension. The methods you master should become part of your everyday routine, and open your eyes to the true meaning of the gift with which you were blessed. Although becoming an empath isn't a disease or a curse, it's controversial and might cause you to feel so insecure that you'll try to suppress it. In anonymous alcoholics or opioids, their motto is the first step towards healing is to admit you have a problem. The same applies to you as an empath; acknowledging that you are indeed an empath and that you are proud of it is the first step towards accepting your gift. While this is a small move, it will make a huge difference, and you will remove a lot of the tension associated with hiding your gift.

It is important that you get enough rest to feel released from the challenges of becoming an empath. The most successful way to do so is to set a daily sleep-wake cycle and do what you can to make sure you have a restful nighttime sleep. You should also take daily breaks for relaxation and deep breathing exercises during the day to relieve yourself of some of the tension that has built up all day. Such exercises will give you prompt relief. Take note that you do not put yourself in constantly excessively stressful situations. It can be hard to avoid them entirely; you should try to avoid them as much as you can, however. If you know you will be in an excessively stimulating setting, make sure you brace yourself beforehand, both emotionally and mentally. This will help you to get rid of all of the tension you feel as a result of the energy that you are surrounded by quickly.

Overall, social media and the Internet are highly stimulating environments. It's suggested that you regularly take a break from the energy released across the Internet. You needn't be in someone's physical presence to consume their energy. It's also recommended you have a daily stress management routine in place. What you do depends on how comfortable you find yourself. You may enjoy reading books of inspiration, having a massage, going to a spa, using aromatherapy, or taking a warm bath.

HERE ARE SOME HELPFUL TIPS TO HELP YOU ACCEPT YOUR GIFT FULLY

APPRECIATE YOUR STATE OF CONSCIOUSNESS

Empaths, since they are distinct, also feel strain. Being different presents many challenges, as the world expects you to abide by its rules and principles. It is easy to take their criticism personally and bear it as a burden when you are misunderstood by others. Being emphatic and a blessing to be physically and spiritually in tune with yourself is natural. I will go so far as to suggest that to survive, it is important that you have this gift because it puts you on high alert when you or your family are in danger.

IDENTIFY THE DIFFERENCE BETWEEN THOUGHT CONSCIOUSNESS AND EMPHATIC CONSCIOUSNESS

The difference between day and night can be noticed since you can see it. Identifying emphatic sensitivity is complicated, so you can't see it. It is something on the inside that is felt and learned. You can begin to see your gift as a blessing instead of a curse until you can recognize this difference. When you know when the mind and its emotions are dominating, you gain self-knowledge. Feelings are different, and you'll feel liberated when you understand these distinctions. This awareness will give you the power to protect yourself from energetic waves, rather than being drawn into it.

TRUST YOUR INSTINCTS

Many of the empaths who awaken to their gifts ignore their gut instincts. Do not do this; it is only your experience that is correct. This doesn't mean you can completely grasp the emotion, or accept it. You may not have full understanding of the situation, but the feeling is real, and you can accept the deeper contact that exists within.

CHAPTER 11:

UNDERSTANDING THE IMPACT OF EMPATH ENERGY

When empaths begin to accept their gift and know they don't have to bring the resources of other people around with them, a natural curiosity about resources sets in. Through your symptoms and interactions, you become conscious of how strong energy can adversely affect you. If that is the case, the energy may also have a positive effect on you. When you've learned how to cope with the energy-carrying tension, you'll be liberated to learn how to use energy positively. It is an exciting journey to learn how energy operates, and it can take you to places in life that you didn't think existed. Many empaths become healers, as you have read; these are the individuals who have learned how to accept their gift, and they know how their energy can have a beneficial impact on others.

In learning about energy, the first step is to understand how to base yourself on various energy sources. This will help you stop getting overwhelmed by the energy you might be experiencing. Visualization is one of the most prevalent grounding strategies. This is where you knowingly imagine that you are grounded; here are some steps to get you started:

- Sit comfortably in a chair and put your feet squarely on the floor with your palms facing upwards. Don't push yourself into a certain position; just let your body relax on the chair. Imagine that a piercing white light radiates from the sun and through the chakra of your crown, leaving your spine at the bottom and then into the center of the earth. Imagine the harmful black energy is being emitted through your hands as your body is filled with white light. You will naturally relax when your entire body is filled with white light, knowing that you are now filled with positive and peaceful energy.

- As a strategy to keep you grounded on the ground beneath you, to release the negative energy that has attached itself to you, and to enhance your empathic gift, you should practice visualization on a regular basis.

- Working with energy confidently will cause you to stop feeling as though you are out of control. It will help you to protect yourself and heal yourself and the people who are put in your path. Ultimately, it will give you the power to regulate the force that is directly impacting you.

There are many things that you can excel in when you learn to effectively handle energy, which is one of the reasons it is so attractive to many. It is your divine right to learn how to navigate this powerful terrain of energy so that you can use it in a way that benefits you and others.

MEDIUMISTIC SKILLS

By tuning into the spiritual energies around that person, a medium uses its intuitive or psychic ability to see into the past, present, and future of the life of an individual. Mediums rely on the existence of a supernatural force outside of themselves to accurately gather knowledge about the person they read. A friendship is made with the deceased in the function of mediumship to convey messages to those who are living. Knowledge is obtained directly from the spirit guides, angels, and the dead.

There are four major Mediumship types:

THE CLAIRSENTIENCE

You sense the feelings and sentiments of people, spirits, animals, and places intensely. In both your heart and in your body, you sense these emotions; you feel the presence of spirits as well. If you have skills which are clear:

- You are very sensitive to your surroundings; you can feel a person's or a place's vibe easily.

- When you go to areas where there are big crowds, you have unexplainable physical or emotional responses.

- All of a sudden, your feelings change when you are around people or when you arrive at a person's house.

- Without them asking you, you know what people feel; you can easily empathize with people.

- The presence of spirits can be sensed.

- You can feel it in your own body when people are in pain.

- You know what people are feeling without them telling you; you can empathize with people easily.

- You can feel the presence of spirits.

CLAIRCOGNIZANCE

Spontaneously, knowledge comes to you; you don't doubt it and believe in your soul that it's 100 percent true. Either this knowledge comes in the form of statistics and facts, or you only know the reality of a case, a girlfriend/boyfriend, or a career path. If you possess clear-cut skills:

- You get the answers to stuff and don't remember how or where it came from.

- You have very inspiring, imaginative, and beneficial thoughts.

- Your mind is never quiet; you always come up with a new idea, especially when you're working on a project.

- You immediately know whether or not anyone is telling the truth.

- In having conversations with others, you tend to use the words "I know."

CLAIRVOYANCE

Before they manifest, you see stuff as images in your mind or as a precognition in dreams. If you are clear-sighted:

- You still have very vivid dreams.

- Are highly creative and spend a lot of daydreaming time.

- Talk often in metaphors.

- When you close your eyes to sleep or during meditation, you can see forms, colors, images, or objects.

- You see sparks of light from the corners of your eyes, sparkly lights, or gestures.

- When you speak to someone, you also use the words "I see."

CLAIRAUDIENCE

Either within your subconscious or audibly, you hear messages. These signals come in the form of telepathic communication for the majority of people, indicating that through your emotions, the spirits can have a conversation with you. With the spirits, you can have a conversation, and they will respond.

If you have such clairaudient characteristics:

- Listen more than you say.

- You are referring to plants and animals, since you think they can interact with you.

- You always feel as if you are the recipient of telepathic data.

- You forget what you said straight away when you give very helpful advice, and wonder where you got such wise knowledge.

- You sometimes hear your ears humming or ringing. Right before they pop up on an airplane, you feel the same feeling in your face.

- When talking to individuals, you use the words "I hear."

They are also attracted to mediumistic abilities because of the intuitive nature of the empaths. This is not an empath's normal characteristic, but that doesn't mean you can't have the gift; because of their openness to the spirit world, it is often easier for an empath to cultivate this ability. If you feel like you are attracted to this field and you decide that you want to improve this talent, it is not something you can take lightly, and finding a good teacher is crucial. Empaths, as you have now discovered, harvest all sorts of energy, whether positive or negative, and it will haunt you if you come into contact with the wrong spirit.

PSYCHIC ABILITIES

Empaths are capable of feeling things before they manifest; the psychic capacity is closely associated with the ability to "just know." Before they happen, you will also experience visions or premonitions. You can not learn to have dreams or premonitions, but if you need to, you can prepare yourself to have them. This gives you the beautiful and strong ability to predict future events. You may not have had any premonitions or dreams yet, but this does not mean that in that talent you may not operate; it may be that you have not yet tapped into it. You will find it simple and exciting to foresee the future, as you learn how to manage this gift.

ENERGY PROJECTION

One of the aspects you may not be aware of as an empath is that you can give energy to humans. You give the person the specific feeling or vibe you want them to feel when you do so. This is an ability used for remote healing, where, although they are not even in their presence, empaths are able to heal others. Others see this as a way to pray for others and to send positive energies and feelings in another person's direction to help them get through a tough time when they can not be there personally. Sending energy is not limited to empath; if they put their mind to it, anyone can do this. When empaths transmit energy, however, the receiver is more likely to feel it because they have a strong connection to the source of energy.

HEALING

Empaths recognize the interaction between energy and humans, which is referred to as an energy body, which can be afflicted with disease or pain. When you're trained in healing energy, you learn how to work with the energy body of your own or another individual to trigger healing to create a balanced body of energy.

CHAPTER 12:

EMPATHS AND SPIRITUAL HYPERSENSITIVITY

Empaths also suffer from hypersensitivity dependent on spirituality; the signs include:

- Your surroundings make you feel overwhelmed.

- Sounds, even though produced at a regular range, are too noisy.

- You often sense other people's emotions.

Nothing fresh is this sort of energetic overwhelm; for many years, the spiritual world has been grappling with it. When more and more empaths chose to disregard their gift, they become less linked to the world, which has led to a rise in hypersensitivity centered on the spirit. Oversensitivity to the energy and noise of people is a normal answer to energy acceleration, you can expect to feel it as you ascend to higher heights in your spiritual growth. You can sound like a radio transmitter picking up a million signals at once when you start to accelerate in the spiritual realm. When a change in spiritual vibration happens, your sense of intuition and your emphatic channels are open, creating a heightened awareness of those around you. Spiritual hypersensitivity can physically manifest, causing dizziness in the third eye, energy hypersensitivity, odors, light and noise.

Metaphysics assume that the body is the spirit's vessel, that the body is not who we are; in our spirit, our individual is borne. We are divine beings living in a physical universe, says Wayne Dyer. Anything that happens in the physical first happens in the spiritual realm; thus, it will manifest in the physical body if there is an imbalance in the spirit. Until concentrating on the physical, metaphysical health counselors often explore the spiritual dimensions of recovery, as it is a spiritual balance that heals the physical ailments.

HOW TO COPE WITH SPIRITUAL HYPERSENSITIVITY

The fight or flight syndrome is triggered, and breathing becomes shallow when the body is stressed physically, emotionally, or mentally. When you start feeling a change in your breathing pattern, you should start practicing conscious breathing immediately. This is where you concentrate your attention on your breath, which will slow down and allow you to relax your nervous system. At the same time, breathe slowly, deeply, and in a rhythm, while concentrating your mind on being able to relax in the situation in which you are. You should always take a brief escape from any unpleasant situation, such as issues relating to family or work. A good way to do this is to excuse yourself, and go to the toilet. This will encourage you to get away from the negative energies, practice, and refresh your breathing techniques.

There are also some methods that you can use for spiritual healing:

PRAYER

Prayer will still offer relief in a daunting situation, depending on what you believe in. The H'oponopono prayer is one of the most thought about and powerful prayers. Here's the story behind it.

For the mentally ill, the Hawaii State Hospital was a facility for those who had committed the most egregious crimes. Because of their mental state, criminals who had committed murder, robbery, rape, or other crimes of such nature were either sent there or to decide if they were sane enough to stand trial. It was a place of little hope, according to one of the nurses who worked there; the environment was so congested with evil and negativity, that even paint did not want to live in the building and did not adhere to the walls. It was all rotting, decaying, repulsive, and scary. Not a day will pass without violently attacking anyone.

The doctors and nurses were bound by fear; when a prisoner stepped in their direction, while shackled by hand and foot, they would walk as close as possible to the walls to keep them safe. Not even shackles could avoid the assaults, however, and so the prisoners were never taken outside unless it was an utter emergency. The majority of the time, workers were absent and would also take sick leave to recover from the depressing and unsafe atmosphere in which they were employed.

A new doctor was employed every few months because the prisoners were unable to treat them, but one day, Dr. Stanley Hew Len joined the clinic. The nurses were not excited at all; they were persuaded that he would be like the others and bombard them with his perceived superior technique that would put the place in order and then depart within a few months when he understood the truth of the situation in which he had himself. They soon realized that something about this doctor was different; he didn't do anything essential, but the world didn't match his personality. Wherever everyone else was sad and frustrated, he'd always been happy, optimistic, and smiling naturally. He would ask for the inmates' files every so often; he never saw them personally, but he would sit in his office and look through their files. To staff members who were interested in the manner in which he wanted to work, he would tell them something he called H'oponopono. Things began to improve in the hospital as the months progressed, the walls were painted, and the paint actually stayed on the walls, which gave the place some energy. The gardens were being pruned, the tennis courts were being restored, and the workers started to play tennis with prisoners who were usually never allowed to go outside. They started to encourage some of the prisoners without their shackles to move about, and the inmates began to take less psychotropic drugs.

The change in the environment was amazing; the workers started coming to work, and where there was once a lack of candidates, there was now a strong demand for workers in the clinic, and they began slowly releasing the prisoners. For about four years, Dr. Hew Len was employed by the clinic; by the time he left, there were only a few remaining inmates who were ultimately housed in another location because the clinic had to close because their services were no longer needed by the prisoners.

It seemed that Dr. Hew Len did not apply any particular procedure or offer any medicine to the inmates. Everything he seemed to do was look at their archives, but with a traditional Hawaiian spiritual healing referred to as H'oponopono, what he did was heal himself. In Dr. Len's own words, "the part of me that formed them was healed." He would feel pain and sadness for them as he sat in his office, staring at every single patient file. Then Dr. Len would use what he thought to heal himself, taking full responsibility for what each patient seemed to be experiencing. The inmates were healing because their doctor took their pain and treated them by himself.

H'oponopono is based on the idea that our own world is created by us; there are no external factors responsible for what takes place in our world. If your boss is bad, then you are to blame. You are accountable if your kids are not doing well in school. The responsibility for world wars, and suffering is yours. The bottom line is that the world is yours and it is your duty to take care of it. Taking responsibility doesn't mean the issues are your fault, it just means you have to repair yourself to repair the situation you find distressing.

Some may agree with this theology, and it may seem totally incomprehensible to others; but if you really want to examine it, you will find the truth is the interpretation of the universe. If you think the world is depressive and meaningless because you want to concentrate on all the negative that affects you, that is how you view the world. If you were to concentrate on changing yourself, you might change that. Two people can live in the same world but, simply because of their experience, they view it entirely different.

So how can you heal yourself with H'oponopono? There are four steps to this concept:

- **Repent**: Say you're sorry for the role you've played in the stuff you consider to be evil or troublesome around you. You can claim as empath that you're sorry for the suffering that the people you've recently met are feeling. Say you are sorry for whatever you feel guilty for; feel guilt and mean it.

- **Ask for Forgiveness**: You may think, "Well, who am I asking?" We all have different systems of belief. Most of us believe in some kind of higher force, particularly empath, and that is who you ask to forgive you.

- **Gratitude:** Say thank you; gratitude has so much strength. If you take the negative off your sight, you'll find that you have so many things to be grateful for. Say thank you for the morning you got up. Say thank you for getting your eyes to see, your nose to smell, your legs to walk on, all of your inner organs in working order. Find something to say thank you for, and keep saying it.

- **Love:** Love is the most strong force in the universe; the words, "I love you" will bring love into your life over and over again. You can say to your cat, your home, your car, the sky, the trees ... I love you! Say it to something that you feel love for.

WATER

During periods of hypersensitivity, water has remarkable balancing and healing properties. It gives inner alignment when overwhelmed with consciousness. By placing a drop of water on your third-eye spot, you can balance the ambient energy. It leads to even more efficient outcomes when you add water that you have energized. Through praying over it, or putting a word on the bottle with the intention of infusing the frequency of words into the bottle, you will energize water. Words that work well, such as healing, calmness, and harmony.

For aura cleaning and for the restoration of energy balance, taking a hot shower works well. Take a shower and imagine the water washing away other people's negative feelings, impressions, and ideas and imagine all the negative energy being sucked down the drain.

MINDFULNESS

It can pull relaxing energy into the body through this process. At the same time, focus on your breath and look at something beautiful like a rose, the sun, or the sky. As if this is the first time you have seen them, you can even focus on the palm of your hands. By focusing on something visual, you can redirect the attention you pay to your feelings.

ESSENTIAL OILS

Essential oils have a calming effect, and the anxiety associated with spiritual hypersensitivity can greatly decrease. The American College of Healthcare Sciences conducted a study in 2014, in which 58 hospice patients were given a daily hand massage for one week using a blend of essential oils. The oil blend was made up of lavender, frankincense, and bergamot. All patients reported less depression and pain as a result of the essential oil massages. The study concluded that essential oil blend aromatherapy massages were more effective for depression and pain management than massage alone.

The following are some of the best oils for treating anxiety:

- **Lavender**

Lavender oil has a relaxing and calming effect; it restores the nervous system, provides inner peace, better sleep, causes a reduction in restlessness, panic attacks, irritability, and general nervous tension. There have been several clinical studies proving that inhaling lavender causes an immediate reduction in anxiety and stress. One study discovered that taking lavender oil capsules orally led to an increase in heart rate variation in comparison to the placebo while watching a film that caused anxiety. The study concluded that lavender had an anxiolytic effect, which means that it has the ability to inhibit anxiety. Other studies have concluded that lavender has the ability to reduce anxiety in patients having coronary artery bypass surgery and in patients who are afraid of the dentist.

- **Rose**

Rose soothes depression, anxiety, sorrow, shock, and panic attacks. A research was conducted by the Iranian Red Crescent Medical Journal in which a group of women undergoing their first pregnancy inhaled rose oil at the same time as taking a footbath for 10 minutes. A second group of women who first witnessed pregnancy also obtained the footbath but without the inhalation of rose oil. The findings showed that a footbath combined with aromatherapy induced a reduction in anxiety in women in the active phase in nulliparous women (a woman who has not yet had any children).

- **Vetiver**

Vetiver oil contains energy, which is reassuring, soothing, and calm. It is also used by trauma victims and assists with rehabilitation and self-awareness. It has a soothing effect, as well. Vetiver oil is a tonic of the nervous system; it decreases hypersensitivity, jitteriness, shock, and panic attacks. The Natural Product Research conducted a study analyzing rats with anxiety disorders and found that vetiver oil was causing anxiety reduction.

- **Ylang-Ylang**

Ylang-ylang has a soothing and uplifting impact; because of its ability to trigger joy, cheerfulness, and bravery, it improves depression and anxiety. Ylang-ylang often soothes anxiety, heart agitation, and nervous palpitations. It is also a sedative which helps with sleeplessness. A 2006 study by Geochang Provincial College in Korea found that using a four-week combination of ylang-ylang, lavender, and bergamot oil once a day induced a reduction in blood pressure, hypertension, serum cortisol levels, and psychological stress response.

- **Bergamot Oil**

Bergamot is one of Earl Grey Tea's ingredients, which has a distinctive floral fragrance which tastes. Bergamot oil provides calming energy that decreases depression, agitation, relaxation causes, and insomnia helps. A research conducted in 2011 showed that anxiety, depression, blood pressure, and heart rate were decreased by the application of bergamot oil.

- **Chamomile**

Chamomile oil is renowned for its soothing influence and its capacity to build inner peace, alleviate fear, anxiety, over-thinking, and irritability. An exploratory research was conducted by the University of

Pennsylvania School of Medicine and found that it has therapeutic anti-depressant properties. It was also noticed by the National Center for Complementary and Integrative Health that chamomile capsules have the potential to alleviate symptoms linked to anxiety.

- **Frankincense**

Thanks to its quiet energy and soothing effects, Frankincense oil is perfect for managing anxiety and depression. It also allows you to concentrate, calm the mind, and deepen your meditation. A research by Keimyung University in Korea found that a mixture of lavender, frankincense, and bergamot decreased pain and stress in terminal cancer patients at the hospice.

HOW TO USE ESSENTIAL OILS IN CALMING HYPERSENSITIVITY

In aromatherapy, essential oils are either swallowed, applied topically, or used.

Here are some ideas for their use:

Aromatherapy

Aromatherapy is a very common anxiety treatment because of the capacity of humans to interpret information by smell; it can induce a powerful emotional response. In the brain, there is a region called the limbic system, which controls memory recall and emotional processing. Inhaling the smell of essential oils stimulates a mental response in the limbic system of the brain, which controls tension and calms reactions such as hormone production, blood pressure, and breathing patterns. You may use diffusers in the bath with the oils, hot water vapor, direct inhalation, a humidifier or vaporizer, cologne, perfume, a vent, or aromatherapy.

Oral Application

Most essential oils can be ingested orally. It is important, however, that the oils you use are healthy and pure. Much of the oils sold have been combined with synthetics or diluted with other ingredients, rendering them unfit for use. Combining a drop of oil with a teaspoon of honey or dropping the oil into a glass of water is the most efficient way of eating essential oils. You may also add a few droplets to the food you prepare. A few drops can be put under your tongue. This is especially helpful since the blood capillaries are located near the surface of the tissue under the tongue, which enables the oil to absorb into the bloodstream rapidly and migrate to the region of the body where it is needed. You may also take capsule-shaped essential oils.

Topical Application

Topical application is the practice of applying essential oils on the body's skin, nails, teeth, hair, or mucous membranes. The oils are absorbed by the skin easily. Because of the strength of the oils, diluting or combining them with a carrier oil such as coconut, avocado, jojoba, or sweet almond oil is important. The blended mixture can be applied directly to the affected area, around the rims of the ears, the sole of the feet, in the water, through a warm compress, or through a massage.

CHAPTER 13:

HOW EMPATHS DEAL WITH INSOMNIA, ADRENAL FATIGUE, AND EXHAUSTION

They also experience a sudden decrease in energy due to the emotional burdens that empaths bring, which leads to chronic fatigue. They will unconsciously give their energy to others when an empath does not stay grounded, healthy, and actively aware. In the company of negative or depressed people, when an empath spends too much time, they carry on their resources, and this may lead to emotional fatigue. That is one of the key reasons they need to spend time on their own as a way to recharge their internal batteries. There is a relation between mind, soul, and body; everything we think and feel has an effect on our physical body. In order to process thoughts and emotions, an empath must have frequent periods of solitude during the day. This avoids mental fatigue, which then encourages them to let go of crushing negative energy continuously. They find it hard to sleep at night if an empath does not do this because their minds are unable to absorb and make sense of the knowledge that took place during the day. This hyperactive mentality causes empaths to get incredibly tired. If the empath can not find solitude throughout the day, it is important that they meditate before going to bed so that they can relieve any feelings with which they have come into contact during the day.

EFFECTS ON THE ADRENAL GLANDS

Negative feelings may lead to terror, anger, anxiety, insecurity, and panic experienced by empath, and they become truly persuaded that something bad will happen to them. These thoughts send signals that generate hormones that release excess quantities of energy to the adrenal glands. Not enough sleep, too much stress, poor diet, bad relationships, and issues with family all have a detrimental effect on the adrenal glands. Like the kidneys, the adrenal glands are shaped but are around the size of a walnut. They are situated in the lower back section, just above the kidneys. When we are under stress, the adrenal glands are of great benefit because they help keep us concentrated and alert, and they improve our endurance levels, which helps us to maintain pressure.

However, when the adrenal glands are excessively activated, they begin to create energy, which is what keeps us from sleeping. The mind and body remain on high alert, causing the adrenal glands to be excessively stimulated and ultimately causing them to malfunction. A lack of energy contributes to a craving for high in sugar foods and refined salt, which easily transforms into energy giving the body an immediate but short-lived boost in energy.

The body actually yearns for salt and sugar. We prefer to feed it, however, with refined sugar and salt that is present in most junk and processed foods. These foods can cause a variety of health problems in excess of quantities. Unrefined sugar is nutritious and can replenish and nourish the adrenal glands in healthy doses. You can feel drained, groggy, nervous, irritable, overwhelmed, and dizzy when the adrenal glands are not functioning properly. You can also experience heart palpitations, high or low blood pressure, cravings for salt and sugar, as well as finding it hard to cope with stressful times.

The adrenal glands are not easily overwhelmed if our bodies are in balance, have a healthy diet, sleep well, and have positive thoughts. Cortisol is a hormone released by the adrenal glands. Our levels of cortisol increase and peak a few hours before daybreak during sleep. This is how the body prepares itself spontaneously for the day, which is called the circadian rhythm. It raises our energy levels so that we are able to work during the day. When the adrenal glands are overworked, even though we've had the usual eight hours of sleep, we wake up feeling exhausted. Throughout the day, we feel exhausted, which then causes our cortisol levels to peak in the evening, making it difficult for us to sleep correctly.

KEEPING THE ADRENAL GLANDS HEALTHY AND PROTECTED

Destruction of the adrenal glands takes a long time, and fixing it would take the same amount of time. But there are some improvements in our lives that we can make that will improve instantly. It is important that we spend time listening to our bodies so that we are conscious at every given moment of how it feels. Which helps us to keep track of our energy levels all day long. You could find that your energy levels fluctuate during the day and that when your energy levels drop the most, there are certain periods of the day. It is imperative that you understand why the adrenal glands are experiencing so much tension. We should ensure that we do not linger in that heightened condition that creates more pressure on the adrenal glands when the root cause of the issue is found.

Meditation is a strong instrument for emptying negative emotional mind and spirit. It also allows us to concentrate on the body, because we are mindful of any physical sensations that arise. Cortisol levels will rise when we feel alone, depressed, and separated; you will battle this by spending time with friends and family. However, if you are the kind of person who likes to spend time alone and you enjoy your own business, isolation times aren't an issue. The adrenal gland can be adversely affected by diet and exercise. During a workout, it is not a good idea to push too hard; your body will tell you when it has had enough, and it is important that you stop at this point, or cause the adrenal glands to produce excess hormones related to stress.

The adrenal glands all induce overwork by eating junk food, missing meals, and hardcore workouts. We should consume an organic, nutritional, and well-balanced diet with the regular protein requirements, with vitamins A, B, and C, in order to keep the adrenal glands in a safe state. You should avoid excessive alcohol and ideally minimize the intake of refined salt, sugar, and caffeine. A positive state of mind leads to healthy adrenal glands, where you feel calm and happy with life and get adequate sleep at night.

WHY YOU SHOULD CUT OUT REFINED SALT

Research performed by the University of Washington's director in Seattle has shown that low levels of sodium cause a decrease in blood volume. The body compensates by triggering the sympathetic nervous system, which releases adrenaline, which activates the response to fight or flight, making sleep difficult.

WHY YOU SHOULD CUT OUT REFINED SUGAR

It can cause disrupted sleep cycles, often from vivid dreams, when the adrenals have been overworked, both of which can cause increased anxiety. Stress and anxiety due to excess cortisol lead to sleepless nights; this usually takes place between 2:00 and 4:00 a.m. The hormone rush makes it hard for us to stay calm and wakes up the body in an anxious state.

HERE IS A NATURAL REMEDY THAT WILL HELP ELIMINATE THIS ISSUE

SALT AND HONEY

With 1 teaspoon of Himalayan rock salt, mix five teaspoons of raw organic honey. Place a small amount under the tongue twenty minutes before going to bed and let it dissolve. The salt and honey combination naturally de-stresses the body by controlling the hormones. This leads to a harmonious, calm, and calming state that prepares the body for deep sleep. Honey and salt also help the body so that you do not wake up feeling hungry during the night.

Many who eat honey and salt before going to bed have confirmed that they no longer experience lack of sleep; they sleep all night long and wake up energized and refreshed, and no longer experience dips of energy all day long. Bedtime anxiety has now been replaced with peace and tranquility in the awareness that they will sleep in a matter of minutes and stay in a sound, smooth sleep.

THE BENEFITS OF RAW ORGANIC HONEY

Honey helps release glycogen from the liver into the brain. A lack of liver glycogen allows the stress hormones cortisol and adrenaline to be released by the adrenal glands. Tryptophan, responsible for the development of serotonin, a hormone that causes relaxation, is one of the ingredients in honey. Serotonin is converted to melatonin when there is no sun, which triggers restorative sleep. Melatonin controls the cycle of sleep-wake, as it acts in accordance with morning and evening. When our melatonin levels are stable, we quickly and naturally fall asleep when it gets dark, and our body immediately wakes up when light begins to invade the room.

We were taught to think salt is bad for the health; this assertion is not entirely accurate. The metabolism is stabilized by a good balance of the right salt. We must have a healthy metabolism, since it is important to make sure that the food we consume is consumed and converted into energy. Salt has anti-excitatory and anti-stress effects, reducing our levels of stress and helping us to stay calm.

We also have a need for salt that doesn't know it reduces anxiety and provides an overall sense of wellness. Sadly, the majority of us will eat processed foods containing refined table salts that have no health benefits when this need arises. When we start eating unrefined salts like Celtic, Himalayan, or Real Salt, we immediately find that our stress levels are going down, our energy levels are going up, and we have a consistent mental and emotional state.

Eating after 7 p.m. is another misconception. Causes weight gain; to support this, there is no empirical proof. There is evidence, however, to indicate that an evening snack helps us stay asleep because the adrenal stress hormone is activated by the brain when we get hungry, which then puts us on the alert for fight or flight.

THE BENEFITS OF HIMALAYAN SALT LAMP

A salt lamp from the Himalayas is a large piece of pure Himalayan salt, with a small bulb inside. It offers a subtle warm glow that enhances the air's consistency. An excess of positive ions is released into the air by cell phones and laptops. As the ions are balanced, a Himalayan salt lamp can make you feel better and produce a sense of calmness and freshness in the air. An ion is a molecule or atom in which the number of the electrons is not equal to the sum of the protons; this gives the atom a net electrical charge negative or positive.

Positively charged ions are also known as cations, and negatively charged ions are also referred to as anions. The mixture of charged negative and positive ions causes them to attach in the atmosphere and travel around.

Sunlight, lightning storms, ocean waves, and waterfalls usually contain negative ions. There are some advantages associated with negative ions, according to Pierce J. Howard, the author of "The Owner's Manual for the Brain." They allow more blood to circulate through the brain, leading to less drowsiness, more mental energy, and more alertness. In the atmosphere, they protect against germs, which cause sneezing, irritation of the throat, and coughing. One in three individuals is susceptible to the potency of adverse ions, which can quickly make people feel refreshed.

The best way to get negative exposure to the ions is to spend time outdoors, especially around water. Small amounts of negative ions are formed by the Himalayan salts. Electronic machines, such as microwaves, TVs, computers, and vacuum cleaners, produce positive ions. They can cause health issues, such as sleep loss, allergies, and stress, and exacerbate them. Negative and positive ions bind together, leading to the positive ions being neutralized by the negative ions. This approach helps to purify the air. Salt lamps also have a gentle light, which is soothing for many people.

Salt is hygroscopic, which suggests that, due to the heat produced from the light bulb, it attracts water to the surface so that it evaporates easily. In humid climates, this is one of the reasons why salt lamps leak water. It carries bacteria, mold, and allergens when there is water vapor in the air. Salt lamps attract both the water vapor and the elements it holds to the lamp surface, thus extracting it from the air. That is one of the salt lamp's most beneficial functions.

A LOW-LIGHT LAMP ALLOWS FOR A PERFECT NIGHT LIGHT

The body is influenced, according to studies, by various colors of light. After the sun goes down, it is recommended that blue light is avoided because it can have a detrimental influence on the circadian rhythm, which disrupts sleep hormones. The majority of light sources emit blue light, such as tablets, laptops, computers, TVs, and cell phones, and most of us spend hours staring at these screens at the end, especially during the evening. Salt lamps offer a warm orange light close to the light radiating from the candlelight, or from a campfire. That's why they are a beneficial source of light, and they can stay on all night without interrupting sleep.

Soft orange hues increase emphasis for those suffering from seasonal affective disorder (SAD), improving energy levels, and relaxed moods. The negative ions also contain elements that improve the mood.

CHAPTER 14:

HOW TO SHIELD YOURSELF FROM ENERGY VAMPIRES

An energy vampire is a person who absorbs your energy; energy suckers and psychic vampires are often referred to as these. Some vampires of energy are mindful of what they are doing, and others are not. Usually, the unconscious are mentally ill or emotionally unstable; they have a dire need for someone with safe and powerful energy to pull life from them. Empaths will normally feel dizzy or exhausted when a vampire absorbs energy from them.

There are also conscious vampires of energy who have been conditioned by negative and dark powers to gather positive energy. They do this for different reasons: gaining respect, gaining strength, boosting their self-esteem, boosting their ego, and for youth or health.

Protecting yourself from energy drainers is essential; here are some techniques to assist you:

DON'T GIVE TOO MUCH

Giving is good as it increases your psychological understanding, spiritual development and personal evolution. It is however important that you replenish yourself when you give; you must master the balance of giving and receiving. When someone gives you something tiny, such as paying you a compliment, receive it with an open heart and say thank you; there's no need to give them back and return with another compliment.

REFRAIN FROM PLEASING PEOPLE

There are some individuals who will want to please everyone. This is obviously not possible; we all have vibrations of varying frequencies. You are going to attract those you're on a common vibration with, and the ones you're going to deflect. When you want to please others, you can be your own energy vampire.

BE WARY OF THE GREEDY PEOPLE

You would be drained by people who are just concentrated on themselves. If you're having a chat with them, they're all talking about what they're doing because they're going to wonder how you're feeling like you're going to be part of everything. At the end of a discussion with them, you will feel drained; limit your interaction with, or exclude certain individuals from your life entirely.

BE MINDFUL OF NEEDY PEOPLE

To get your attention, desperate people do anything and all. They ask for your support and advice constantly, but never submit it. These guys are going to waste your time and drain your resources. Train yourself to know when you're dealing with those people and reduce your contact with them.

LOOK OUT FOR DRAMA QUEENS

These people aren't hard to identify as they are often involved in some sort of problem. They are continuously bombarding you with texts, phone calls, and text messages about the current tragedy in their lives. You'll not have many resources left until you know it. It's important you don't waste your time engaging with such people because they are going to kill your energy field.

CLARITY

Don't waste time with people beating around the bush, get right to the point. Shut them down when a person is too negative; when a person continues to act with the same patterns and then requesting your help, shut them down. If someone asks you to do something for them, and you're unable to do so, just say that. You don't have to be mean, you just have to be firm and let people know what your limits are so they don't exceed them.

HERB SMUDGING

Smudging requires the burning of herbs to produce a bath of cleansing smoke for protection, purification, and healing purposes. Palo Santo Wood, also referred to as Holy Wood, is a type of sacred wood used for purifying, medicinal purposes and to expel evil spirits by the indigenous people of the Andes and the shamans of Peru. Cedar, sage, and pine can be used for smudging.

CRYSTALS AND GEMSTONES OR GEM ELIXIRS

To protect against emotional distress, risk, psychological assault, empath and oversensitivity, quartz crystals, tiger eye, amethyst, tourmaline, obsidian, and onyx are all used.

ORGONE

Orgone has many functions, including the formation of a safe energy field covering your atmosphere and your aura and the deflection of harmful energy. They are often used as a shield to deflect toxic pollutions and frequencies from electromagnetics. Four orgone protectors should be positioned in the four corners of your home to protect against harmful energy and to ground spiritual energy. The Safe Orgone Amulet provides protection from psychic attacks, negative vibes, mental pollution, and evil eye.

THE CANDLES

Candles do away with bad/negative energy from your home. Also, they are outstanding for purposes of manifestation. For self-protection, dark blue, red, and white candles are good colors to use.

INCENSE AND RESINS

To purify the atmosphere of homes and landscapes, incense made from natural substances such as frankincense, myrrh, sage, sandalwood, and musk are used.

FOR BATHS

Add 1/2 cup of sea salt to your bath; this will cleanse harmful energy that after being in the presence of such individuals has attached itself to you. Steep a teaspoon of clove or basil into a cup of boiling water, strain the herbs out, and apply them to your bath; these herbs are known for their properties of cleansing and protection.

PROTECTION CHANTS AND PRAYERS

Using strength, zeal, and dedication, any chants or prayers will work as long as they come from the heart.

CHAPTER 15:

EMPATHS AND HOW THEY FUNCTION AT WORK

You'll be facing specific organizational problems as an empath. Everyone wants a job that suits their talents and personality, but before taking a role, you need to take extra precautions because a toxic work environment will easily make you mentally, spiritually, and physically ill. So, as an empath, how do you choose the right sort of job and flourish at work?

ASK FOR A TOUR OF THE WORKPLACE BEFORE TAKING UP A JOB

Ask if you should take a tour when you go for an interview if someone hasn't already offered to show you around. Pay attention to the facial gestures of the staff, their body language, and the way they speak to each other. You can easily guess if the business is toxic. Respect your gut instinct and avoid workplaces that involve a large amount of negative energy unless you are in dire need of funds. Pay careful attention to the lighting, the levels of noise, the amount of clutter, and the desk layout. Ask yourself if you could be working comfortably in such a setting, from both a physical and emotional viewpoint. A high salary can be an attractive one, but first must come your health. Even if other people are telling you a job is too fine a chance to pass away, trust your instincts. You have the ability to make a positive difference in the workplace, but you do not have the responsibility to risk your mental and physical wellbeing if you do so outside your comfort zone. When choosing the best career for you, never feel bad.

USING YOUR GIFT AS A SELLING POINT

Empaths are, by default, not show-offs, and the idea of selling yourself in a work interview can be sufficient to make you feel queasy. But think of it this way—really, the empathic skills are an increasingly important asset in the workplace. We tend to equate the business world with a sort of cut-throat attitude, and even the public sector, where everyone is trying to outdo each other and fight for the best positions and the most money.

Our culture, however, is increasingly conscious that the only way forward is to take care of one another and our world. In building a more caring environment, we still have a long way to go, but in general, we are beginning to recognize the advantage of a balanced work-life balance and the significance of cooperative working practices rather than a dog-eat-dog mentality. You can use your gift to help push this transition if you feel up to the challenge!

You know that life and work are something more than position or pay. Your gift makes you ideally suited to positions that include abilities to listen, settle disputes, and mentor. Dr. Judith Orloff, a therapist, author, and empath, maintains that empaths carry their professional positions with zeal, outstanding communication skills, and leadership abilities. When an interviewer asks what you can bring to a job, don't hesitate to provide examples of times these talents have been demonstrated.

WORKING ALONE VERSUS WORKING WITH OTHERS

Although you have strong leadership potential, a position that requires extensive day-to-day interaction with colleagues and customers may prove to be too exhausting, especially if you are not yet confident in your ability to deal with negative energy and toxic people. When applying for a role, be honest with yourself. If it means working as part of a busy team with little chances of recharging during the day, think carefully before applying.

Many empaths are well suited to operating inside small organizations for themselves or taking on workers. It might be too stimulating to function in a big office or noisy atmosphere—and that's great! We all have different needs and abilities, so don't allow someone to make you feel bad because you can't do a "usual" job. As an empath, the idea of having to deal with colleagues, management team members, and clients will easily overwhelm you.

Working alone, on the other hand, will result in social isolation if you take it to extremes. For example, if you plan to run a small business from home, be sure to arrange some time at least a few times a week with family and friends.

You not only need to cultivate your relationships, but it's also useful from time to time to obtain an outsider's viewpoint on your work. You may get so wrapped up in a project often that relatively minor issues tend to take on a life of their own. It helps you to take a more rational perspective and to help you come up with new ideas by talking to other people.

IF YOU'RE IN AN ENVIRONMENT THAT DRAINS ENERGY, ASK FOR REASONABLE ADJUSTMENTS

You can't expect your employer to redecorate the office just to suit your tastes or to fire an energy vampire, but you can politely ask them if a few minor changes will be important to them. For example, if directly over your desk there is a harsh strip light, you might ask if it would be possible to turn off the light and instead use lighter, gentler lamps.

Experiment with white noise or other sound recordings intended to cause feelings of relaxation and emotional health if you work in an atmosphere in which people speak loudly. Try captured sounds in nature, as these are also calming for empath. On YouTube or specialized noise-generating sites like mynoise.net, you can find lots of free tools. If possible, for at least a portion of your workday, listen to natural or white noise using noise-cancellation headphones.

You may also make additions and improvements which do not require your boss's permission. For example, as a way to combat negative energy, you can put crystals on your desk and set aside a few minutes per day—even if you're extremely busy—to ensure your desk is free of unwanted clutter. Choose a relaxing scene or color as your screen wallpaper if you work with a computer. Frame and keep a picture or uplifting image on your desk. Look at it for a few seconds, if you need a constructive dose of energy.

If you enjoy your job, but would like to spend less time with others, consider asking your boss if you can work a few days per week from home. This will give you a respite from the energy of other people and helps you to take a break at any moment. Working from home comes with the luxury of creating an atmosphere that best suits you. For instance, you could add a water feature on your desk or play natural background noise during the day without fear of getting your colleagues to ask intrusive questions.

LOOK OUT FOR ENERGY VAMPIRE

In your personal life, if you come across an energy vampire, you usually have the option of cutting ties with them, or at least restricting how much time you both spend hanging out. Sadly, when you are forced to work with them, this isn't the case.

Here's where boundaries come in. From the beginning of your professional relationship, you need to respectfully but firmly assert yourself. Don't be drawn into tiny office gossip, and don't embrace toxic people's invites to socialize outside of work. Take advantage of your best self-defense energy skills and always place your well-being before professional responsibilities.

Empaths who want to work in helping careers, whether with other people or animals, need to be mindful of their work's effect on their energy levels. For instance, if you work as a counselor or therapist, it may leave you drained, tired, and even depressed to talk to a person who is going through a very sad or stressful time in their life. Be sure to allow yourself to be grounded in a few minutes between clients or meetings, and arrange plenty of time outside of the job to relax and nurture yourself.

CREATE BOUNDARIES BETWEEN YOUR WORKPLACE AND YOUR HOME

It's a smart idea to formulate a schedule that establishes a simple dividing line between your professional and personal life if you work outside your house. You are open to taking the negative energies of others with you as an empath. Not just about the issues you face at work, but also those of your colleagues, managers, and clients, you might find yourself worrying about. You'll quickly become overwhelmed, nervous, and depressed unless you learn how to "turn off."

Be mindful of the change between work and home when it's time to finish up your work for the day. Develop a routine that helps you to turn your attention to personal desires and emotions immediately instead of those of colleagues and clients. For example, when listening to a specific soundtrack or piece of music, you might want to spend the final five minutes of your workday in meditation or tidying your desk. You might get into the habit of messaging them just before leaving work or on the way home if you have a friend or relative who often increases your energy levels.

FOCUS ON HOW YOUR WORK WILL BENEFITS OTHERS

Changing your career or working in the area of your choice isn't always possible. Try to approach your career with a different attitude if you are trapped in a career that is not right for you, and are in no position to make a shift any time soon.

You have a gift to support people, as an empath. They not only benefit from your encouragement, but you also get to soak up their positive energy as well. It is a win-win situation, really! As long as it does not leave you feeling too exhausted, try to find ways to lend a hand to someone else and give emotional support.

For instance, if one of your colleagues seems particularly stressed, take the initiative and ask them if they would like to talk to you about anything that is bothering them for five minutes. Often, just giving a listening ear will turn around someone's day! Or maybe you can provide a more realistic type of support. For instance, on your coffee break, you could offer to take everybody's mail to the mailroom. Service and kindness acts allow you to find meaning in your work, even when you hope to change careers in the near future.

CHAPTER 16:

HOW TO NORMALIZE AND MAINTAIN YOUR EMPATH GIFT

Now that you've learned how to accept your gift and maximize it, the next step is to normalize it. This includes learning how to make the gift a natural part of daily life. You will no longer need to worry at this point about how you plan to react or how you want to use your gift, you will only be able to use it and reap the benefits from it. In thinking about tapping into your gift, there will be no need to make any effort; it will become like the air you breathe.

The process of normalization is a vital part of moving completely into your gift as empath. It will free you from thinking about being an empathic, because you are able to do it regularly now. You never have to worry again that your gift has some kind of hold on you, because you now know what to do when things get out of control. When you want to, you will be able to tune in and out of the electricity.

You will never become drained of all the emotions you used to feel; you will only feel the emotions and energies you want to feel when you are normalized. You won't take energy from other people anymore or experience an immediate negative response to the energies you're exposed to. Once upon a time, because of negative energy, you may have lost your temper or been tired and drained. You could have avoided crowds, public areas, certain individuals, dinner parties, family events, and house warming parties because you knew you would leave a tired, overwhelmed, and exhausted feeling that could last for several days. During that time, you've been perplexed as to where these feelings come from, resulting in you feeling confused and annoyed.

You no longer encounter these negative emotions now that you have grown used to life as an empath. You can walk in and feel energized and inspired in a room full of new or familiar people. You no longer consume other people's thoughts and energies; you are always able to read their thoughts, so they do not have the ability to keep you hostage any longer. You know how to ground yourself and deflect the thoughts that are not helpful to you, energy, and emotions.

PRESERVE YOUR GIFT

The preservation and mastery of your gift are two entirely different methods. When you have mastered your talent, you find it easy to live in harmony with it, and you have normalized it, as discussed above. However, don't get relaxed after you've entered the point of normalization, because now you need to preserve your gift to make sure you don't go back to the early stages of discovering that you've been empathic. In order to keep your gift, there are many things you will need to do. This process will allow you to live with your gift in perfect harmony.

CHECK-IN REGULARLY

It is important that you check-in on a regular basis in order to retain your gift. You should be doing this at least once a day, but you really should be striving for twice a day. First of all, the best times to do so are in the morning and before you go to bed. This will encourage you to focus on the things that have had the most day-long effect on you. In the morning, you are able to remember leftover memories you mistakenly held on to. In our dreams, much of what binds itself to our minds also comes to life; you can then let these emotions go and get on in peace and harmony with your day.

Before going to bed, it is a good time to check-in, so the experiences you have had during the day will be fresh in your mind. You will be able to detect how you have been affected by these encounters and release them so you can have a quiet and restful sleep.

DAILY MEDITATION

The perfect time to meditate is as soon as you wake up in the morning, just before bedtime. But make sure you don't make a habit of meditating until you fall asleep because this can have a detrimental effect on your practices of meditation. It can leave an impression on your unconscious mind that causes you to equate sleeping with meditation, leading you to fall asleep throughout the morning and during the day during your meditation hours. Meditating gives you the chance to use your resources to relax. You don't have to feel like you're in control; there's no tension, and at that moment, you can enjoy your energy.

DEEP BREATHING

It's important that you relax regularly, but you should make sure your breathing follows a certain pattern at the same time. By reaching a state of rest within your body, deep breathing helps you to relax fully. Breathing in for 4 seconds, holding your breath for 6 seconds, and then breathing out for 8 seconds is a healthy breathing exercise that you should try. This will assist in removing any extra air from your body. You can imagine some negative energy or tension leaving the body in the air, at the same time as taking deep breaths.

Deep breathing is an excellent way to concentrate and easily achieve equilibrium within yourself. If you ever find yourself struggling with your grounding exercise, start your breathing deliberately. This will help you recover full emotional balance and return to your power core. It is recommended that you practice deep breathing every day and whenever you are in a distressing situation.

DELIBERATE GROUNDING

A significant part of standardizing your empath skills is that you frequently ground and protect yourself. The grounding method helps you to periodically remove unnecessary energy and go back to your core deliberately. On autopilot, you can never stop retaining your energy, or you can fall out of alignment very easily and become unbalanced. And when you've learned to master your skill as empath, you'll always find you get into situations where you're consuming other people's resources.

CHAPTER 17:

NURTURE YOUR OWN ENERGY

Empaths might wrongly feel responsible for the energies and emotions of other people. Second, because empaths can experience other people's energies and feelings so deeply, then it's easy to feel as if the next step is to try to help them. And helping is often the right next step, but it's a move that should always be taken carefully. Note that you need to have extremely clear boundaries as an empath. In this chapter, we will cover empathically specific self-care techniques that help you to maintain those boundaries when you are tempted to feel responsible for the energies, and emotions of other people.

The second explanation empaths may feel guilty for or want to regulate other people's energies and emotions is a kind of self-defense or self-protection. Empaths may subconsciously assume that if they can calm down someone or make them smile, then they won't have to experience second-hand any of the difficult or intense energies or emotions of the other person.

The solution can act as a temporary remedy, but for the parties involved, it just makes things worse in the long run. It's important to note, for empath, that you should only have control over only your own emotions. And then emotions are meant to be felt more often than commanded. You are taken away from your core, from yourself, and from your control by attempting to exploit, keep, or handle the feelings of someone else. Empaths can be incredible sources of emotional support for loved ones, customers, colleagues, and everyone else with whom they come in contact. But your unique ability to turn up emotionally and energetically to others depends on the balancing act of first appearing to yourself and remaining consciously grounded in your own body. That you do primarily through your practice of self-care. Taking good care of yourself is the number one priority and allows you to love others even more. We'll explore mindful ways to cultivate your own energy in this chapter!

ALIGNING WITH THE FORCE OF GRACE

It is grace in motion when beneficial individuals, opportunities, tools, or experiences turn up for you right when you need them. Grace is a divine, sustaining power that often operates in your life. You can actively increase the amount of grace moments you experience, and activate this energy more fully whenever you want. Alignment with the energy of grace is an ideal way to take care of yourself, whether you are facing a particular challenge or just want additional help. Here are a few strategies for aligning energies with grace.

1. Think of the world as a place of magic and love. Very rough, stressful things are happening but note that miracles are happening too.

2. Look at the bright side of the case, find the silver lining, and look forward to the present and the future.

3. Using a mantra of gratitude, such as "Unexpected blessings for me still turn up."

4. Expect grace and second chances.

5. Be compassionate as much as you can to anyone.

6. Keep open to new perspectives, entities, and possibilities and stay flexible.

7. Say your words frankly and strive to remain optimistic.

While you identify ever more with the force of grace, here are a few things to look out for.

1. Don't dismiss feelings that challenge you yourself. You may be really depressed or upset about everything that has happened, and still, be optimistic about the future, or concentrate on the current silver linings.

2. Be hopeful but be practical too. Remain had grounded on a situation's reality.

3. Take responsibility and, when you can, take action.

4. Learn from the past, but continue looking ahead and note that it can be different and better for the future.

I witnessed grace in motion several years ago as I was searching for an apartment in Manhattan. My quest initially lasted two weeks and was very disheartening. I felt apprehensive and defeated. Nevertheless, I had just been turned on to the power of positive thinking, so I thought, "Ok, let me try and change my mindset and my aspirations." I started thinking stuff like, "I'm a nice person and a good resident, and everybody would be fortunate to have me live in their house." Over the past two weeks, my energy had been anxious, rushed, and closed off, so I relaxed purposefully, opened up, and slowed down. I met a lovely real estate agent within days, and the first place she took me to was my dream apartment, in a brand new house, in a sought-after neighborhood, just blocks away from a beautiful park. The cost was staggeringly affordable. My husband and I spent thirteen years living there, and we were reminded every time we stepped through the front door that miracles were possible. Take one circumstance that has been challenging and modify your attitude and your approach through the recommendations in this exercise to fit more carefully with grace in your own life. Note how this changes your energy to one that is calmer and more optimistic, and watch for outside world changes too. Let others feel good even if they don't. If a loved one, or the outside world, is going through a tough time, it is okay if life still feels pretty good in the emotional and energetic woods of your neck. Remember that:

- You don't need the permission of someone to feel your positive emotions. Celebrating and savoring whatever is going on in your life should be part of your self-care routine.

- Taking on someone else's difficult feelings won't help. Currently, that would actually make things harder for you both.

- Empaths are better suited to helping others because they take excellent care of themselves. It is bad self-care to take on others' energy and emotions.

If someone else is in a difficult position, but you aren't, try the following:

- Ensure you practice focused support. When you are helping them, send someone your full attention, then take your attention elsewhere.

- Put your help to time limits. It's all right to note the moment when a friend is on the phone venting to you.

- Seeking someone else with whom to share your happiness.

- Compassionately and conscientiously honor the suffering of a loved one—or of the universe. Step up your advocacy, make a donation, make dinner for others, or simply tell others you care about.

How you remain healthy is to let yourself experience wonderful experiences. Savoring and celebrating are healthy cares for oneself!

ESTABLISH A CHECKLIST FOR INTIMACY

Empaths can bond very quickly with others, so empaths can sense how other people feel or what they need very easily. It is a beneficial and lovely opportunity to communicate easily with others, but it also has a daunting side. You may get too close too quickly and end up hurt, realizing later that you didn't know the person well enough or long enough to become so transparent and vulnerable.

Rapid intimacy is not always a negative thing. Often a potentially dear friend gets out of the blue into your life right when you desperately need that kind of friendship. In some work cases, such as when you're new to a job but can easily distinguish what the disposition of a manager is like or how you can contribute to the current team in a specific way, this empath to get close easily can also be very useful. Empaths, however, should be vigilant of this phenomenon.

Refer to the following checklist if you easily become acquainted with a new acquaintance, extended family member, coworker, lover, or someone else. Using any of the following questions, you may also build a customized checklist while also coming up with your own.

1. How does this person treat himself? Do they seem to have a strong sense of affection for themselves and a positive method of self-inventory?

2. What is the factor for drama in our relationship? Have we had intense fights before, or have I already doubted the relationship?

3. How long, days, weeks, or months have I known this person?

4. Does it feel like we have a connection with the soul or a deeper bond?

5. Do this person, and I have any mutual friends or acquaintances?

6. How much of the person's history do I know?

7. Has that person been given the chance to turn up for me in a meaningful way or have my back? If so, how is it that they did?

8. Does this person attempt to make me accountable for their feelings?

9. Does this individual make me feel frazzled or exhausted, or do I feel more grounded and relaxed by their presence?

10. Gives the person my own room for me?

11. Does this person care about my health and happiness genuinely?

12. Why is this person talking to me? Is it courtesy and respect?

13. Am I in this person's relationship because I feel like they need me, or because I get something that nourishes them in my life?

14. Is it hard for me to develop emotional boundaries with that person?

15. Did I secretly wonder if, at this particular point in our lives, this person may not be the best match for me as a friend or lover or colleague? Or would it seem we met at the right time?

16. Is this person normally supportive of my hopes and dreams?

17. Is the natural energy of that person suited for me, or does it feel a little too strong or a little too mild for me?

18. Does this person seem versatile or open to change if something isn't working in our relationship?

Note that you or the other person are not intended to judge the questions on this list. The answers will simply help you to grasp the complexities of your current link with them.

PRACTICE RADICAL SELF-LOVE

Empaths may be vulnerable to internalizing other people's critical views on themselves. You can feel the feelings of the other person intensely and deeply, especially if someone is really angry at you or really disappointed in you. It can be harder to engage in experiencing energies to get the eagle viewpoint of your higher self if you are already in an emotionally heightened and vulnerable position.

Radical self-love and self-acceptance are antidotes to being too negative and excessively judgmental about yourself. Use the following self-love strategies for harmony when you are with yourself in a difficult environment, or use them as positive self-care at any time.

1. When you catch a glimpse of yourself, smile, wink, or gaze into your eyes in the bathroom mirror at home and say "I love you!"

2. Find a good, happy image of yourself as a child, frame it, and put it somewhere you will always see it. Remind yourself that you are still part of this lovable kid.

3. If you're angry with yourself about the past, close your eyes at the moment of the painful occurrence and picture yourself. Send the younger version of you, your unconditional love in silence and give a quick, wise pep talk.

4. If you've been frustrated or regretted an action, get your journal and write down five ways you've improved or wanted to improve for the better because of this experience or five lessons you've learned from that experience. Five is a number correlated with big life changes that are optimistic.

5. Serenade yourself by putting on and singing a tender love song to yourself. Singing will open up the chakra of your neck, which allows you to convey and process feelings.

RECOGNIZE INTENSE, NEUTRAL OR MILD ENERGY

Having a system of classification for different types of energies may help empaths become more conscious of how others' energies may influence them. Energy can have several subtle layers, and it can be individual or collective energy. For example, a national disaster could generate an atmospheric energy of sorrow, but healing and connection still have undercurrents. We will categorize this energy as intense. Some people or locations may also be idling with different energies, such as a quiet town described as sleepy (mild energy) or grounded (neutral energy) therapist. Here's how you could be influenced by each form of energy.

1. Intense energy has the potential to impact you in a broad way. If a friend is on top of the world with a naturally powerful intensity, they can be a pleasure to be around as you open up to experience some of the sparkle! If the same friend is irritated, to have strong self-care boundaries, you will want to engage in witnessing energy.

2. Neutral energy, like a blank canvas that allows empaths to tune into themselves, can be nourishing. You can find that your office has a comforting, neutral background energy when there are no stressful deadlines, and people are happy in their positions.

3. Mild energy can be a nice break—or it can get dull. With a balance of energies, life is best, and each empath will have distinct preferences and tolerances for mild and extreme energy at distinct times. Energy assessment as severe, neutral, or mild.

People, environments, and groups may have a baseline or natural energy, and dramatic energy fluctuations or gradual changes can also be experienced. For humans, including empaths, it's natural to be a fascinating, fabulous combination of different energies.

GOSSIP DETOX

You will try to stop engaging in (which also means listening to) celebrity "news" and family or office gossip for two weeks, for this exercise. Diplomatically bow out or redirect conversations involving gossip, without gossiping or causing unnecessary drama on the guy. Wherever you find yourself drawn to stories about others during this two-week period and afterwards, ask yourself:

1. Will the knowledge have some direct impact on me? If a coworker gossips about how your manager changes teams, the answer might be yes. If the gossip is about the divorce settlement of a manager's personal information, then the answer is possibly no. For the next two weeks, that's the sort of gossip you can stop.

2. Will this data help me communicate with myself better? Maybe a friend is sharing a story about their sibling, and how this sibling is going through so many major changes at once that it makes them feel ungrounded. If you are still struggling to remain focused when facing several huge changes, this "gossip" will help you get more in contact with your own feelings, and it is perfect for this exercise to listen to some of the information for a brief period of time. If, however, you catch yourself reading about the rehab stay of a celebrity only because you're bored at work, for the next two weeks you can find something else mindfully and lovingly to fill your thought. You will hopefully build a different relationship with celebrity news during this conscientious gossip sabbatical, as well as family and office gossip, and be better able to distinguish when hearing or reading about others is safe and when it is toxic, constantly clogging up your sensitive system.

RELEASE SOMEONE WITH LOVE

When you care deeply for someone, keeping them close to your energetic heart is natural. But when a relationship changes or ends dramatically, or keeping someone close becomes unbearable, it's therapeutic to release them. This release occurs on an energetic plane, which literally shifts the intimacy level between you and the other person. Since empaths are so energy-sensitive, reducing the link of energy between you and another can have incredibly positive effects on you and even the other person on the physical plane! Nevertheless, you don't have to let the other person know about this exercise or connect with them—so it's a perfect way to break up or build conscious distance from somebody who's still in your life.

The practice of lovingly releasing others will help you do many healthier things, such as:

1. Process more effectively or rapidly through the traumatic feelings.

2. Forgive the other person or embrace him, or find happiness for yourself.

3. Pass on and seek closure from a partnership.

4. Bring into your life new relationships.

5. Have a more neutral experience and less triggering when you communicate with that person.

For any partnership, try this ritual. (Seek psychiatric assistance if the other person makes you feel physically or mentally unsafe.)

1. Build an aura of healing—play sacred music, light a candle, keep your favorite crystal, or burn some incense.

2. Imagine being gentle and enjoying the energies around you. Image the energy as rose, gold, or green, heart-related colors, and healing. Take deep breaths as this force is washing you over.

3. Close your eyes and imagine a heaven for healing. It can look like a lovely room with fluffy pillows to sit on and beautiful sunlight streaming through the windows. Or it could be outdoors, like a field of softly swinging wildflowers in the wind where you can lay a comfy blanket and sit down. Like the tower chamber in a large castle lined with beautiful tapestries, your healing sanctuary could look very special. Take a moment, and let the specifics fill in your intuition and imagination. Anytime you like, you can visit this healing sanctuary. If you have a spirit guide, love someone who has passed on, or an angel with whom you would like to function, call them in to be with you.

4. In your soothing sanctuary, imagine yourself. Then think about who you want to release. You can imagine writing their name on a piece of paper, or you can put a picture of their face on it. Give the silent message to their soul that you wish them well and expect them all the best. Tell them that you're freeing them from their bond with you, and tell them something else that feels correct.

5. Remember what emotions exist in you (with your eyes still closed, relaxing in your sanctuary of healing). Let yourself feel them, and after you close the ritual, make a note to return to them.

6. One last time, take in the details of your healing sanctuary and say farewell to it for now. Open your eyes slowly. To complete the ritual, take some deep breaths with your hand over your heart.

You could come up with a lot of emotions or intuitive hits about potential realistic action measures. Get help from loved ones or healthcare practitioners, and recognize that releasing someone is a process that typically can not be accomplished in one ritual. As emotions come up in the following days or weeks around this subject, let them. Think "I'm releasing them with love" when your mind returns to this person, and feel in your heart the gentle, peaceful energy of that purpose.

CONFRONT OTHERS WHILE YOU DEFEND YOURSELF

Empaths often shy away from confrontations because they are unwilling to consume the demanding energies and feelings that can be brought out of others by confrontations. But it is a necessary part of enacting change to question others often, or freely disagree with them. It helps you remain close to yourself, respect your feelings, and practice self-care by telling someone else how you really feel or what you really think. It's also a way for other individuals to genuinely turn up for their benefit. Next time you need to confront someone, try the following empath-friendly conflict strategy.

1. Process your thoughts in advance. Share the raw ones with someone you trust, like a good friend or counselor.

2. Think of what you want to say and what in the conflict you intend to achieve beforehand.

3. Using the empathic abilities to respond to what might be the emotional experience of the other person. You might get the intuitive knowledge that a romantic or business partner is frightened or overloaded with work about the future, and that's why they're so rude to you recently. With healthy skepticism, look at any observations you receive. You may or may not be right after all. This move is intended to help you see the other individual more compassionately or holistically and remind you that there may be other problems at play that have nothing to do with you.

4. Just before you confront this person, take a couple of minutes to enter observer mode, and engage in witness energy. Relax and get grounded, maybe by meditating, listening to the sounds of nature, telling yourself a supportive mantra, or picturing a ball of golden or blue light around your body.

5. Tell the other person how you feel and whether you want to be as cool and diplomatic as possible. Offer them room to respond, and really listen.

6. Pay attention to any new intuitive experiences or feelings you feel about the situation after the conversation.

While it may inherently be more difficult for empaths to challenge others, it is an ability worth honing and a life factor worth making peace with, both for your personal and professional lives. If it's difficult for you to challenge others, keep trying, get more help or instruments, and practice radical self-love in the process.

Empaths, because of their desire to communicate with others and understand where they come from, are also natural diplomats and negotiators. An empath may also be effective at conveying someone else's viewpoint to a wider community—like a family, a group of friends, or a people-filled workplace. However, an empath may confuse being a negotiator with having to manage the emotional reaction of someone else—or speak to someone else out of their emotion or reality if it is especially difficult for others. In addition, empaths among loved ones or colleagues can be respected for their negotiation skills and then called upon to behave so frequently in this capacity that it becomes exhausting.

There are individuals at home or work who can hardly be in the same room unless I am there to de-escalate stuff.

If you have replied to many of the previous prompts frequently, you might be trying to control the energies or feelings of other people, or working as a shadow rescuer. You could often find that your effort to control other's unhealthy acts or uncomfortable feelings simply escalates matters—as well as drains you. Now, answer the next set of prompts sometimes, occasionally, or rarely: Being the negotiator between people at home and work is one of my strengths: people know it, people admire me for it, and when I have the emotional reserves and physical energy, I genuinely enjoy this job. And when I perceive what someone else thinks or wants from others, I make sure that I still express my own feelings and desires.

By communicating and voicing it, being more open to your own emotional experience will actually help you become more open to other people's emotional experiences too. Actually, this will boost relationships! Empaths should not repress their own feelings, or attempt to contain other people's emotions.

CHAPTER 18:

HOW TO SUPPORT A YOUNG EMPATH

Now, as an empath, you know how to take care of yourself and how to best use your gift. If you have a youthful empath in your life, however, it is important that you also understand how to help them. Children with this skill frequently face crucial obstacles, but when they come to grips with the fact that they are different from their peers, your encouragement will make all the difference.

It's hard to be an empathic kid, but young people have so much to give our society, and they ought to be appreciated! Dr. Michele Borba, psychologist and empath specialist, claims adolescents today run low on empath. They are, in truth, just half as caring as those of previous generations. It's obvious that young people with empath have a lot to tell their colleagues.

HOW TO SPOT A YOUNG EMPATH

Empathic talents come from birth, and young empaths have the same strengths and needs as empathic adults. However, since children have less experience of understanding and communicating their own emotions, they can manifest their empathic nature in a different way.

Empathic kids usually tend to play alone or in the company of either one or two good friends. In reality, they derive more pleasure from talking and playing with older kids and adults than those of their own age. It's not because they think they're superior to their classmates. Rather, the uncommon maturity of a young empath means they are on the same page as older ones than themselves. They can report feeling isolated or disconnected from people of their own age.

With their uncanny capacity to hone in on what others are thinking and feeling, an empathic child can surprise you. For instance, while cooking dinner for the family one evening, you could feel worried about an incident at work. Your empathic child may walk past the door of the kitchen and discover immediately that you are upset about something that has happened during the day. Well, they could give you a hug and ask you to tell them specifically what or who made you sad.

It is crucial that you strike a balance between respecting their gift and overloading them with knowledge that is not necessary. If you're frustrated or angry, denying it will teach your child that they can't trust their instincts, which can instill uncertainty and self-doubt.

On the other hand, too much information may not need to be revealed, as this might cause them undue distress. A small child, for example, may not need to know anything about a medical condition or an attack. In certain situations, a clear acknowledgment of the situation and the emotions that go with it would suffice. Do not lie to your child and keep age-appropriate conversations going.

REVEAL THE REAL MOTIVES BEHIND TEMPER TANTRUMS

Before chastising a young empath for poor conduct, consider deeply. Yes, they might literally disobey you because they're a bad kid, but they might also behave in response to excessive stimuli in their environment.

Take the situation from the viewpoint of a toddler. As an empathic adult, if you find yourself bombarded by too much noise or light, you can usually make excuses and leave. A small child, sadly, has less autonomy, and also has no choice but to suffer. They can either freeze up in an effort to defend themselves, which is why empathic children are often called "shy," or they can try to regain control of the situation by creating their own noise and chaos!

If you suspect that your child is an empath, don't be surprised if, from time to time, they unexpectedly act out. If they often have meltdowns or tantrums, it is time to look a little deeper. Just think like a detective. Are there any triggers which predict "evil" behavior reliably? Take the concerns of your child seriously—trust them if they tell you they don't like heavy light or smells!

Let anyone else who cares about your child know that they are an empath, or that your child is exceptionally sensitive and needs a few slight changes, whether this definition is unfamiliar to the individual concerned. For example, if they are attending a daycare center, you can let the workers know they are prone to get distracted during high-energy games and might take some time out to calm down.

You should not yell at a young empath, use cruel punishments, or resort to offensive methods such as name-calling in any circumstances. These techniques are damaging anyway, but they are likely to inflict long-lasting harm when the child in question is an empath. If you're losing your temper, immediately apologize. Take full responsibility for the behavior.

BUILD A FRIENDLY ENVIRONMENT

Make sure that an empathic child has a safe space they can call their own, and encourage them to escape when they need to relax and recharge their batteries for some time alone. Even if you have family or friends over, if they need to spend ten or twenty minutes in their room, then leave them. At the end of a busy day, empathic kids can take more time to wind down and get ready for sleep. Their nervous systems are easier to activate than those of normal kids, and it is impossible that just asking them to get into bed and close their eyes would result in a good night's rest!

To help them relax, it's a good idea to schedule a bedtime routine. You may, for example, prepare them a bath with soothing essential oils, tell them a common story about bedtime, and inspire them to focus on the best things that happened that day.

HELP THEM TO PLAN FOR THE HARSHER REALITIES OF LIFE

Caring for an empathetic child can be heartbreaking at times because when they know how much misery there is in the world, their gentle, kind hearts are easily bruised. Often, they are more likely to hurt feelings when an argument breaks out in their social circle. An empathic child may be trying to understand why other kids seem to harm each other when they can never act so cruelly.

Attempting to protect a child from pain is natural and normal, as a parent or caregiver. Sadly, while it can succeed in the short term, in the long run, you will be doing them a disservice. Later, as they come up against the harsh realities of the world, an empath who is not taught how to work with their gift and control their feelings early in life is at risk of depression, anxiety, and uncertainty.

You can't fix the world's problems but, you can keep your child's communication lines open. Give them the opportunity to talk about it when they pick up on signs of stress and emotional distress, be it at home or in school. Encourage them to completely express themselves—after all, emotions are there to be felt. Early on, teaching them coping mechanisms is much better. This empowers them because they know that almost everything life throws their way can be treated.

GIVING THEM REALISTIC APPROACHES THAT THEY CAN USE

So how do you empower a young person with the resources they need in a harsh environment to thrive?

Firstly, teach them how to meditate, and the importance of taking at least a couple of minutes of grounding each day. Children are more open than adults to new ideas, and you probably won't have to waste a lot of time and energy encouraging them to try it out. Why not allocate time per day for joint meditation? Not only can this help them develop a healthy habit that will last a lifetime, but it will also strengthen their relationship.

Secondly, help them learn to verbalize their thoughts, give them a name, and understand how the feelings of others have a direct influence on their moods. Emphasize that selecting good friends who are generally happy is crucial, and spending time with individuals who leave them feeling energized instead of down.

Empaths of all ages, sadly, are favored targets for energy vampires and abusers of all sorts. Teach your young people how to create boundaries, set their own relationship expectations, and walk away from people who want to hurt them. Make a point of reminding them that if they want or need advice about how to treat a toxic friend or bully, they can still come to you. Practice saying "No," and use role-play to rehearse how your child is able to get rid of tough circumstances.

Model the type of conduct in your child that you want to see. Do not deny your own emotions, spend time when you're overwhelmed, and draw firm lines when others want to take advantage of themselves. Children are keen listeners, and for guidance, they look to their parents and caregivers.

Take action to fix the issue if you live in a home where two or more people often get into fights. In their living environment, young empaths pick up on stress, and this can lead to extreme psychological and physical illness. In certain cases, family therapy may be appropriate.

TEENAGER EMPATHS

For almost all, the teen years are tough, and they pose unique challenges for empath. To seek approval from their peers, to break away from their families, and establish their own identities is natural and common for adolescents. During this time, it is common to experience heightened, tumultuous emotions. Normal adolescent issues, however, can escalate into long-lasting psychological chaos for an unsupported youthful empath.

A real problem for teens is peer pressure. They may agree to take part in risky behaviors such as drinking, smoking, underage sex, and reckless driving in their attempt to gain the approval of their peers. Fear of peer rejection can also push mature empaths to put themselves at risk. They have to recognize the value of strict boundaries for their own safety, and say "No." If they have not mastered this capacity by the time they reach puberty, don't worry. To understand, it's never too late.

For the first time in puberty, depression, anxiety, and other mental health issues frequently emerge. This suggests that not just their own mental health issues but also those of their peers may have to be discussed by young empaths. They would feel compelled to give a listening ear or shoulder to cry on, as instinctively caring individuals. This is an admirable response, but the young empath will soon feel overwhelmed by the sheer force of the emotions of a friend.

It's best to provide a straightforward, nonjudgmental approach. Educate your teen about the difference between natural teen feelings and mental health issues in teenagers. Teach them how to identify mental illness symptoms within themselves and others, and teach them when and how to get help. Bear in mind that they do not feel comfortable talking to you, so reassure them that if they want to seek advice elsewhere, you would not be offended.

If they help a friend, praise their compassion but, at the same time, stress the value of maintaining personal boundaries. If your buddy drains his own emotional reservoirs, it's time to point them in the direction of professional assistance. Reassure your teen that their friend can not be expected to "save" and, often, calling on a qualified adult's resources is the safest option to take. To sum up, the early years of a life of empath are vital to their health as adults. Young empaths soon understand that they have unique skills. If the adults around them are not helping them, an empath may feel isolated or even isolated from others. Fortunately, they will come to appreciate and enjoy their incredible gift with gentle encouragement and nurturing.

CHAPTER 19:

KEEPING YOUR EMPATH SPACE CLEAN AND UNCLUTTERED

Empaths, should be specific about their emotional and energetic connection to clutter, which can be different for each empath. There's a beautiful furniture store across the street from my office with high ceilings and lovely plants and candles, an empath I knew who worked in a huge open-area office with several other workers and piles of documents, books, and other items on almost every surface told me. Often, I'm going to sit there on one of the couches and decompress on my break. A different empath may be unaware that they're using clutter on their desk as a kind of energy shield, and need to find a better shielding solution.

Many empaths are irritated by the clutter, overwhelmed, and unnerved. With these tips, keep your room and your resources tidy, safe, and uncluttered:

1. Declutter – Try the famous Marie Kondo method of asking, "Does this item spark joy?" when you examine your belongings. Give yourself some time to think before you start throwing items away or donating them, if you're not sure.

2. Be emotionally present with yourself as you declutter. Some clutter may make you feel more emotionally comfortable or serve as an energy shield; powerful or nostalgic memories may emerge from clutter.

3. First, tackle the more apparent culprits. While the stuff tucked away in "junk drawers" or closets is draining, even more draining is the clutter you can see out the entire time.

4. Arrange items left with shelving, colorful baskets, or boxes which look tidy.

To start decluttering, select one manageable spot, so the task is less daunting. Pace yourselves!

BE INTENTIONAL ABOUT YOUR DECORATIONS

Physical objects produce those energies and feelings in humans, like the painting you love that hangs in your hallway or the rug you hate in the living room of your father. Empaths, who are hyper-perceptive and notice more about physical environments, want to decorate their environments with colors, artifacts, works of art, and pieces of furniture that generate positive energies and emotions in them.

Your energy can be drained by a room you find deeply aesthetically displeasing. Many empathic clients tell me there's a room they've been trying to beautify in their home or workplace, but they can't find the time or energy. This room then becomes even more of a drain of electricity. What room in your life most needs an empathic makeover? To decorate with purpose, take manageable, inexpensive measures. Any things that should be kept in mind are:

1. Less is more, because an empath can generally be bothered by a clutter (unless it is unintentionally used as an unhealthy shield of energy). It's not important for you to spend money on a lot of things.

2. Make the space your own authentic style—regularly adjusting when your style changes—so spending time in this space can be a way to re-ground your energy and link it back.

3. Different colors, fabrics, designs, and objects will alter your energy while decorating and affect your mood. Does the vibes test have a room that encourages positive vibes?

Some empaths sense old energies around things, maybe from the spaces they have occupied beforehand. Clear an object's energy by saying a blessing over it, putting the object in a bowl of floral petals, leaving it in the sunlight (be careful not to cause damage) or moonlight, smudging it with sage smoke, or just giving it a gentle clean.

CREATING COMFORTABLE ENERGY

In a given space, you may want to build cozy electricity, because:

1. You are either mentally drained or healed.

2. You're going through transitions or adjustments and feeling vulnerable.

3. Physically, you get upset, and you want to calm down.

4. You're with other individuals and want to create an environment that facilitates relaxation and emotional intimacy.

YOU CAN BUILD MORE COZY ENERGY THROUGH

1. Making the room feel smaller. If you have a wide backyard, at one corner of the porch, build cozy energy.

2. Having everything you need close by, such as holding a book, your reading glasses, and your tea on a side table, so you can snuggle into your setting.

3. Cultivating an environment of kindness and abundance. If you are entertaining others, serve pleasant snacks and drinks—anticipate what your guests want so they feel well-nourished, such as setting out special choices for people with food sensitivities or people who don't drink alcohol.

4. Creating pillows and throw pillows for physical comfort. Keep soft blankets of varying weights for different seasons, and lay a blanket over your body (some empaths enjoy weighted blankets), stack small pillows in your lap, or place oversized pillows on either side of you. Physically snug feeling will calm sensitive people down.

For any mood, many empaths could find cozy energy an ideal go-to. When you're with others, cozy energy can give empaths a lovely balance, where they don't feel under- or over-stimulated.

CLEAR THE ENERGY OF YOUR SPACE

Spaces, like humans, still carry energy. You may want to conduct a ritual to clear up your energy if the room you are in feels overwhelming, stagnant, or energetically cold and uninviting. You can also clear up the energy of a room:

1. After you physically clean it, as part of your routine maintenance of a room, such as a home or office.

2. Because the room is new to you, and you want to clear from previous tenants some old electricity.

3. Since everything in the room either looks energy-efficient or funky.

4. Since there have been a lot of strong emotions swirling around the room lately, such as parties, intensities relevant to work or school, or battles.

5. As part of your own grounding of your energy work.

Clearing the energy of a room may obviously be very effective, but in some cases, it is not recommended. Do not try to use energy clearing, for example, to:

1. Get rid of a wandering spirit. I've had clients telling me they've been trying to use the sage to flush the odd force they thought was a ghost out of their houses, and it can actually make things worse. These energies must be directed toward a better, more healing, more caring position.

2. Avoid addressing or coping with a greater issue. If you are battling with roommates or family members with whom you live in a house, energy clearing will certainly help sweep away the old energy and put more uplifting, new energy in. But it's not going to fix the underlying problems happening magically. However, this ritual will allow you time to communicate with yourself to tune in to your intuition on what is really going on in these relationships and the next best steps.

For this energy-clearing ritual, you will need to pick a cleansing tool: smoke (from incense in a small pipe, a sage stick, or incense in a wand shape), water (I prefer to use an aromatherapy spray), or sound (from a bell, tuning fork, rattle, or singing pipe).

1. Find a time when you can spend 20 minutes to an hour or so alone in space (depending on the size of the space), and do a physical light cleaning of the space beforehand. Choose a smoke, water, or sound instrument you want to use as your cleaning tool. Stick to the sound or water tools if you think smoke or smells will

annoy you or anyone else who uses the room. Everyone is effective!

2. Get grounded before the ceremony. Sit in room, and enter a state of meditation. Decide what energy you want to put into space, and find a word for that energy, such as compassion, healing, harmony, inspiration, pardon, goodness, mercy, or grace.

3. Take your energy clearing tool, and walk around the room slowly. If you are dealing with smoke, wave the stick or wand of the incense, or keep the bowl so that the smoke travels around and fills the room. Attach your singing pipe, hit your tuning fork, shake your rattle or ring your bell and let the vibrating sound echo. If you have water, spray your aromatherapy in the air and let the mist float. Reflect softly on the energy you want to create—feel it in your body, say the word aloud, or focus quietly on a mantra, like "Peaceful, caring energy lies here."

4. Note where it feels heavier or thicker for the electricity. The energy around your desk may feel heavier if you're in a home office because you've been working for long hours or worrying about a project. If you've just hosted a big party and everyone has gathered in the kitchen, you might find that there's more energy. Spend more time until the focus feels lighter in these places. Clear each room's corners, where the energy can get trapped, and the middle of larger spaces, where the energy can radiate.

5. Make sure that all instruments of smoke are fully extinguished, and close the rite with a prayer or blessing in your thoughts or aloud.

CONCLUSION
Part One

Now that we've explored many of the attributes of empath, you might find that even though you had not previously considered the possibility, you think of yourself as an empath. You can also find you are not an empathic person, but you do classify as a very empathic person. It's important to take steps to ground yourself, either way, and make sure you shield your energy from any factors that could be detrimental to you. You can also use the above tips and tricks to start tapping into your intuition, and the gifts you get from being an empath. Being an empath, as you've read in this book, helps you to have a strong sense of inner intuition that allows you to pick up on even the most subtle energy shifts. This also proves to be an immense blessing, as you can excel in things like healing powers, manifestation, and even various clairvoyant practices.

Hopefully, you've learned how to become more in tune with your own energies and thoughts by reading this book. While becoming an empath helps you to be very skilled at picking up on other people's energies and feelings, the most important thing is to learn how to apply this to yourself. To discover how you can shield your own energies and feelings from those of other people, you must concentrate on looking inwards. Doing so will encourage you to more effectively apply your empathic gifts. This form of personality is always seen as a blessing, but it can be daunting, and it seems as though it comes with many setbacks. With all the constant over-stimulation that you might find yourself susceptible to, particularly with social media, you might find that you can never really recharge your batteries. The continuous stimulus you find yourself receiving from social media, news, and various social interactions can be particularly draining to empath, and you need to learn how to protect yourself from these stimulators.

It's understandable to feel exhausted, but you can take several different measures to ground yourself and concentrate on redirecting your focus, as we've mentioned. The trick to preserving your own energetic dignity is to concentrate on channeling it into yourself and concentrating on prioritizing self-care and boundary setting so as to prevent the inflow of toxic energy you may otherwise ingest. You should reflect on the talents that come with being an empath, too.

Instead of allowing yourself to be caught up in the energy issues you face, concentrate on applying your intuitive gifts instead. To pull practically everything into your life, you can use the resources of manifestation and meditation. This is a gift! Since you're an empath, you'll also find this ability comes to you very naturally. To concentrate your attention on your unique, energetic gifts, you can use the resources outlined earlier. Through meditation and nature, remember to concentrate on grounding yourself. By doing this, some of the feelings of being out of control that empaths may sometimes encounter can be avoided. This will encourage you to channel your energy into what, like improving yourself and your intuition, really matters.

In order to prevent yourself from being stressed out and exhausted, we must ensure that we maintain a healthy balance of self-care in our daily routine due to the propensity to become overstimulated too quickly. Recall concentrating first on recognizing feelings and energy before responding to them. Empaths also find it difficult for them to respond instantly, or even not to know how to react, which can lead to many problems in their relationships. This can also result in an emotional overload, which can cause problems in various areas of life. However, when you empower yourself to heal your energy and work through any pent-up emotions, you will find that you can thrive as an empath.

There's a lot more to being an empath than you've read in part 1 of this book. It's just the tip of the iceberg here. Your journey has just started, and to deepen your understanding, you will continue to develop in your gift, meet others, and read more. It can also feel like a curse when you are unable to control your gift; after all, who wants to feel continually tired, unwell, and exhausted? It can be hard for you to handle at first, but you can ultimately learn how to use it to manipulate and enrich your life as you learn to accept and have control over your gift. You can also wish to use your gift to change others' lives. Many empaths make use of their abilities as a profession, and others tend to be more secretive. It's up to you to do whatever you want, and there's no right or wrong way to use your gift. The most important thing is that you realize you're not insane, there's nothing wrong with you, and you're able to live a happy and safe life.

It is crucial that those who do not understand your gift do not offend you because it really is not their fault. Unless the person is an empath, it will be hard for them to understand. People will criticize you and accuse you of being over-emotional and fragile, which is not incorrect, but it can be hurtful when it is said in a demeaning way. It is crucial that you learn from these comments to protect yourself from unnecessary energy.

I hope you now have a greater understanding of your gift and accept every part of it so that your life becomes enriched every day.

I wish you all the best in your journeys!

Part Two

INTRODUCTION

The following chapters will address what psychic ability is, the four forms of intuition, and the resources required to help you cultivate your own capacity for negative powers for psychic premonition, healing, and security. It also contains guidance to contact the Spirit Guides, Psychic protection, Energy vampires, how to declutter negative energies, Guided Meditation, Mediumship, Telepathy (also known as Guardian Angels), and how to practice exercises to develop your psychic empath gifts.

You will learn how to perceive the psychic and spiritual signals you are receiving from others and from the spirit world and how to visually and energetically read the people's auras. The aim is to begin at the beginning of what is potentially a long and fruitful journey to discover and reinforce your psychic abilities by offering useful and comprehensive ways to practice "flexing your psychic muscle." This part further discusses psychic development exercises to help you on this new journey, the pros and cons of being a psychic empath, and lots more.

CHAPTER 20:

WHAT IS PSYCHIC POWER AND HOW CAN YOU DISCOVER YOUR INTUITIVE TYPE?

Psychic powers in real life aren't necessarily like what we've grown up watching on TV. Psychics don't get a vivid flash out of anywhere into the future, like a little movie playing in the eye of their eyes, just in time to alert the subject of the vision, so that they can change their fate-not just the stuff of Hollywood is the ability to feel what the future holds. Although it's a lot more subtle than the way it's presented on TV, it's more of heightened intuition.

Today, everyone has intuition, but for various reasons, some people's psychic intuition is greater than others—the most common is that they don't practice it much. They generally don't believe in intuition, and as a result, don't listen to it or can't sense it. It may also be due to emotional blockage or trauma that leaves you unable to tap into your psychic channel and properly concentrate your energy. Therefore, in a person's subconscious, it never grows and remains unused and inactive.

See, your intuition is like a muscle; you must continue to use it and practice it with it to evolve into true psychic ability. If you have grown up in an atmosphere where you have been encouraged, as it were, to trust your "sixth sense," you are more likely to have a greater psychic capacity. However, for all that was brought up by the world's skeptics and/or if you're a skeptic yourself, there is good news! Even if you have not had this early exposure and permission to grow your gift, that doesn't disqualify you from attaining psychic power. Let's get started for those of you who need a bit of a spiritual workout!

One question people, who may be more in contact with their instincts sometimes ask when they feel that something is wrong is: am I just nervous and suspicious, or is my feeling of suspicion legitimate? The trick that generally works to bring your sense to the bottom of the doubt and if it's just paranoia or a true premonition is: if you experience a sudden foreboding flash or any sense that something is about to go wrong. Then it's gone—that's your intuition! Heed the feeling, and listen to what it tells you about what it warns you about. It may be critically necessary. It will not last long, though, do your best to understand it while it is there; you can even write down how it feels. If you get a sensation that something is wrong and really can't stop worrying about it all day to the point that you're over-thinking it and over-analyzing it to try to find out what it means to how you can fix it to the point that you're very worked up because it just won't go away—in this case, it's most likely just paranoia and not a genuine spiritual prediction. It's easy to say when it's fear because the emotion just won't leave you alone.

Another indication that this is a psychic premonition will be a kind of tingling sensation. In general, psychic premonitions are often followed by a tingling sensation in your brain, usually on top of or between your eyes. They don't always come with this feeling, but the odds are that if whatever you think you feel is followed by a tingling in your brain, then it's pretty fair to say it's a hunch.

After a psychic premonition, you might still feel very tired or low in energy, but this may be due to anxiety, as worrying and agonizing over something will take a mental toll and make you feel depressed during the day and afterward. Therefore, this isn't a sure way to say whether it's a premonition. Still, psychic premonitions make one feel exhausted, particularly for beginners, as they don't know yet how to use the universe's energy for support.

Using only your own energy reserve is not necessarily the safest way to go about psychic practice. It is limited (since opposed to that of the infinite universe) and can / will be drained very quickly. If you have a premonition from nowhere (i.e., getting a premonition even though you were not trying to get one), it would not leave you an option to be supported by the energies of the universe, so if you are setting out to do a psychic reading, it is vital not to use your own limited energy source and try to read and receive unassisted premonitions.

When you start to awaken your psychic abilities, you'll start to see some changes in your life. This is a sure sign that you are on the right path and that your skills are developing. Keep an eye out for something that's out of the ordinary that you find about yourself or whether people tell you to look different. This is likely because you have started to awaken your instincts, you vibrate at higher frequency!

One certain indication of this is vivid dreams. You'll find that the more you're in tune with yourself and talents, the more vivid your dreams will be. If you're someone who seldom dreams or barely recalls your dreams (and if you do, it's just vague pictures and feelings), you're going to find an improvement in your dreams, and you're going to be able to remember them more vividly. This is because your subconscious is more opened up and less blocked once your psychic abilities have been awakened, so the dreams flow more naturally. In dreams, you can receive psychic messages as well. It also increases your vitality, awareness, and relation to the spirit world to be more in tune with your instincts, which can show itself to you in your dreams now that your mind has awakened more.

You can also experience a higher incidence of headaches, along with vivid hallucinations and tingling sensations. Please consult a doctor if you do, just to be healthy. It may be a sign of the straining of your mental capacities and being tired of the psychic work you have been doing. The amount of energy you have to use to communicate with and reflect on your instincts and the psychic world is great. Even though you tap into the universe's energy, it can still be a huge strain and a burden for a beginner psychic's brain to bear. However, don't be afraid—headaches should begin to dissipate as you advance, improve your skills, and become more concentrated and stronger. Eventually, as you become more comfortable and in tune with your instincts, psychic readings will become like second nature—and while they are likely to be always tiring, headaches can subside unless you do a particularly challenging reading or a reading that takes a tremendous amount of energy, concentration and time. If they do not end, please speak to your doctor again about your symptoms. For all the signs, aches, and pains associated with a psychic reading, etc., this is crucial to note. Being healthy and having them tested is always easier since psychic talent is only one potential explanation.

You will also find that now that you are on the road to psychic consciousness, the other senses become heightened. If you've found that while you're watching a film, you no longer need the subtitles switched on, your pallet has improved slightly, your eyes seem brighter than normal, or colors become more vibrant, you're more receptive to certain fabrics. You can easily pick up and pinpoint scents, this can be due to your enhanced psychic ability. After all, you increase your sixth sense; it's only normal that the others also increase in capacity. Now, even though your psychic skills are growing, if you get discouraged because you still need your glasses, just note that being a psychic is not a cure for anything. It will not immediately let you see with 20/20 vision or give you a refined pallet; it can only raise your senses slightly; that's all. It's just a sign of mounting force.

The stronger your pulse gets, the more your psychic abilities start revealing themselves. The stronger your motivation and vibration are, the less time you want to spend with negative people or doing negative things. Don't be shocked if your eyes are opened to the negativity and bad behaviors of some of the people in your life while on your psychic journey. This is an entirely natural aspect of the psychic journey, and you may end up feeling the need to exclude certain individuals from your life or avoid performing certain harmful things in which you have engaged. Unnecessary drama, rudeness, gossip, harmful behavior, and so on are examples of things you can begin to have a strong desire to avoid or stop. This is not to suggest that from time to time you can't indulge in your favorite reality TV show, or cut a friend out of your life because they're dealing with addiction or because they're having a bad day and get mad at you or are pessimistic in the sense that they're depressed and maybe struggling with depression. However, you don't want to be surrounded by people who remain relentlessly negative and drag others down with them. Suppose it feels right for you and eventually gives you satisfaction and empowers you on your journey. In that case, it's best to eliminate these individuals (as kindly as possible, without being disrespectful or meaningful about it, be respectful and compassionate if you think they owe it) or avoid doing these things that bring negativity into your life. Negativity is very exhausting to the non-psychic, so you can imagine what it is doing to someone likely to be very vulnerable to other people's feelings, thoughts, and resources. This is why psychics are better off avoiding negativity.

An increase or development of the psychometry for new psychics is also popular. Psychometry is when you can feel the energy or background associated with an entity by merely touching it. Ultimately, you may also have premonitions associated with the object. However, when you are still a beginner, you may only find that you can feel a certain object's energy, sometimes not consciously. This is fairly popular in antique shops. Brushing against an old silver mirror, locket, jewelry piece, or any old heirloom may, obviously, for no reason, bring you a curious feeling of nostalgia, but this may be due to the past of the piece or the owner of the item.

Maybe they were given the item by the love of their life, who then died or abandoned them or who may have been forbidden to see. This will clarify the sense of longing that is associated with the piece. It typically happens with older objects or objects that have been through a lot and have been through a lot by their current or former owners. It can be clothing items, jewelry, paintings, furniture—even when entering a home; many psychics can sense the energy associated with it and its history / old owners. If you move out soon and go looking at an open house, to get a sense of whether the house is right for you, also take into consideration the place's electricity. Run over the doors, tables, and furniture in any room with your hands.

This should give you a fair idea of whether or not negative energy is abundant, or whether you / whoever you are moving with and the house will be a good energy match. When you enter a home, you will always hear about people's hair standing on end and feeling a sense of evil or bad energy, and then finding out there was a murder or some other horrible incident at some point. This is because, by psychometry, they absorb the energy of the room. People with more developed intuition and psychic skills are more likely to collect energy, so if you start to sense something like this when you contact them, it's a good sign that you're on the right track.

THE FOUR PSYCHIC INTUITION STYLES

Now that we're talking about what your psychic intuition feels like and some indicators that your powers are emerging, let's take a look at and describe the various forms of psychic intuition:

- Clairaudience
- Clairvoyance
- Clairsentience
- Claircognizance

You may not have used these words before, so here is a short rundown of each of them.

Clairaudience

This is when it feels like someone in your head is thinking explicitly. This is more of a brief response to a question or guidance, which shouldn't sound/feel harsh or discordant, not in the same way as people with certain mental disorders. The word "Clair" means simple, and "audience" means hearing from "audire," so you are "hearing" these signals psychically, although it usually is inside the mind. It can sound identical to or close to how you hear people talking in dreams when you have a conversation in your head. These sounds and messages may come from your spirit guides or from the spirit of someone who has died in your life. If you have ever seen someone go on TV to a psychic medium, or maybe you have accompanied someone once to try and reach a deceased loved one, and the medium is going to ask them the meaning of a certain word or sound, they are likely to receive it through clairaudience.

Clairvoyance

It is when you see things that have psychic meaning in your mind's eye. "Voyance" means vision, that is, direct vision. Try examining it the next time an idea pops into your mind, almost out of the blue. It may mean something that comes up in your life in a symbolic (or rather literal) way, or it may describe something that you have been thinking about or wondering about. Clairvoyance isn't going to be a very clear flash into the future where you can see exactly a thing that's going to happen in your mind like a movie-like watching it on TV shows. In your mind's eye, it will be a slight picture or "vision." In the past, you may have had clear-sighted messages without understanding it! Colors, numbers or letters, words, pictures, or photographs of people, things, animals, locations, or something symbolic maybe some examples of what is classified as a clairvoyant message.

The Clairsentience

(Clear feeling) is perhaps the most prevalent of all four. It is when you believe as something will happen. This is clairsentience if you've ever heard anyone use the expression "I can just feel it" or "this doesn't feel right." Clairsentience is also referred to as your instinct or your "gut feeling." Another factor of clairsentience is the ability to sense others' feelings. You could feel a wave of sorrow until your boyfriend gets into the room, and then they tell you that their mother is dead. You could be on the phone with a friend who has a broken right leg, and you notice a brief pain in your right leg, even before you know they've broken it. You can see your pet and unexpectedly burst into tears, overcome with sorrow for no apparent cause, and your pet dies within a week. There are examples of clear-headedness.

Claircognizance

(Clear knowledge) When your intuition allows you to work out something that your logical brain is unable to do, you may be stuck on. If you're caught in traffic, for example, do you risk taking the upcoming exit to get out of it and take the backroad, or will that end up taking more? You decide to wait inexplicably, and traffic has cleared up quickly, and you are on your way. That is clear-sightedness. If you've ever heard anyone say, "I just know," and they don't have any proof to support their certainty or expertise, but they end up being correct—that's experience.

How can you say if you just have an ordinary idea or a psychic message? Sometimes the signs and premonitions can be very subtle. Still, the way to tell is if something (image, sound, feeling, certainty) suddenly pops up in your mind with absolutely no connection to what you were suddenly thinking. This is possibly a message from the psychic and not a feeling. These psychic signals are often very powerful, not a little afterthought in the back of your mind. Often, though, they are quieter messages, so it's always better to try to closely examine it for something that falls into your mind unprovoked-it might have some psychic meaning.

If you just take a closer look at the next sound, picture, feeling, or thinking that springs into your mind unbidden, with these four psychic communication channels, you might find some relevant psychic significance to it. The message(s) will help you obtain knowledge, receive correspondence from the world of the spirit (spirit guides, passed on to loved ones, etc.), or show premonitions or predictions that the other five senses can not. You may have already read this list and honed in on one of the four that you feel more related to or that you think one of them would likely come more easily than the others. In the past, maybe you've used one or more of these, whether or not you knew it at the time. You may have already noticed that, for one, you have more talent than the others.

That's probably the one you're going to be best on and the channel you're going to receive the clearest, most powerful messages, at least for now. I don't say you can't train and consolidate with the other styles. For instance, many psychics started naturally talented at clairvoyance and receiving clairvoyant messages. As they practiced, they gradually became more powerful at clairsentience and perfected it, which became their strongest intuitive medium. This is just one case, but it shows that you're never stuck in just one situation or skillset with just one choice! But, as your best skill, if you want to hold the one you have a knack for, then by all means. Note, emotional power is like a muscle!

Every psychic has a different way of manifesting their strength and intuition, and it's also connected to who they are and what kind of person they are. Everybody has one of four psychic personalities, irrespective of ability. You are either intuitive metaphysical, intuitive physical, intuitive emotional, or intuitive mental. So, how can you figure out what kind of person you are and what fits your psychological abilities? Well, each one expresses itself differently, and you should look at those attributes associated with each form to help you discover the one you identify with the most and which one seems to be more like you. There is no official exam, but in the following paragraphs, each psychic personality is described—and hopefully, you can get a sense of what one suits you.

Physical intuitive people are the ones who have deep attachments to important objects, and psychometry (sensing things by touching physical objects) typically comes naturally. They are the ones that are most likely to use items, such as tarot cards, crystal balls, palm reading, or tasseography (tea leaf reading) to ascertain things about a person or the future and to do psychic readings. When it comes to sensing energy, depending on physical presence or moving their hands close to an object or individual, they are very simply hands-on to get a sense of the items. This makes them the ones most likely to be attracted to the art of psychic healing, or those who typically have a natural talent for the practice. Often they are homebodies and love to arrange their houses, furniture, and decorations according to their interests. Their house is not just a room for them to eat and go to sleep at night, it is their outside world temple and haven, and it showcases a piece of who they are. They spend a solid amount of time at home and have plenty of clutter around the house and drinks. They still completely enjoy spending time and grounding themselves in nature.

The analysts are mental intuitive. They will repeatedly ponder things over, turning them over and over in their heads before they find an answer for something before they create an outcome. They always make sure they take every little detail, review, and double review into account. They never want anything to skip, and they are not major risk-takers, nor are they spontaneous. Mental intuition is more likely to be clear-sighted or clairaudient and to receive psychic signals in their minds through imagery or sound, as they spend much of their time here. So to say, they prefer to "work in their mind" and can go with only the company of their own thoughts for hours on end, only thinking. When they sit down to do a reading for others, they may need the most data and ask for the most information. The logic, reason, and ego are what they live by. They are the ones who make their way through everything. They usually have a strong ability to concentrate and remain focused on what they are doing while working on something, whether it's a psychic related activity or otherwise. They also appear to have very scholarly interests, even if not always.

For spiritually intuitive people, meditation is very important. The harmonious harmony of their energies between themselves and with the universe is crucial. They are quite conscious of spiritual unbalance and can feel it very painfully. Unless they meditate or find a technique for inner harmony and calming to put them in place again, it can make them irritable and feel "off" and discordant. They are less grounded in this world than the other styles and can be characterized as the sort of "getting their heads in the clouds," with a propensity to dream a vivid day very often. Their minds are always roaming around, and they can have a difficult time concentrating on a mission, like psychic readings and/or connections.

In most cases, they are most related to the spirit dimension, who receive or are visited by spirits from the spirit realm, sometimes with a latent psychic force. Most often, they met who died and passed over. Mediumship is always something that is attracted to metaphysical intuition. Aura reading, healing of energy, mediumship, and receiving psychic messages by dreams are all activities that come naturally for the spiritual intuitive in most instances. With subconscious signals, they appear to have very vivid dreams. They may have an affinity for travel as well. However, they do need to be cautious as they are vulnerable to addiction and escapism. Also, they are most likely to worship some kind of deity or higher might.

Emotional intuitives are those who can interpret or feel the emotions of others with the greatest ease. This can often feel like a burden to them as they feel bombarded by other people's feelings and just want to shut it out, particularly for novice psychics / intuitive who are still working out how to turn "off" and "on" these kinds of energy signals. For this reason, they can prefer tiny groups to big ones and enjoy their alone time. They are the classic introverts, partly because being alone at home for them serves as a kind of sanctuary away from all the different energies swirling around the world. They can relax and tune in in this place, not absorbing strangers' various feelings in public. They are, as the name suggests, often very emotional and sensitive individuals. Due to their exceptionally high empathy and ability to feel what others feel, they are identified by many as empaths. They express whatever emotions anyone might have, beyond simply compassion. These individuals have a natural predisposition (clear feeling) to clairsentience. Their high empathy and appreciation of other people's diverse viewpoints make them at heart-friendly to people. They want to make everyone happy and always try to support people. They are the classic personality of "shoulder to cry on." However, it is very important that they do not support this need and that others please take over. They need to be careful not to take advantage of individuals, as is often when other more negative individuals assume that someone is empathetic / emotionally intuitive. When the emotional intuitive is not vigilant, pessimistic, cruel, and deceptive, individuals can energetically drain them dry. They must at all costs avoid that sort of human! It's important for them to understand that they have to stand up for themselves, say no, and take their own time. Instead of using logic, they make choices based on how they feel. They're thinking with heart, not brain. These individuals are natural storytellers, so in occupations such as authors, singers, poets, and artists, you can also find them. You'll also find them inclined to do psychic healing work, similar to spiritual intuitives, because of their selfless disposition.

Hopefully, these brief explanations gave you some insight into what might be your intuitive form, but keep in mind that these are just simple outlines, stereotypes into which individuals can fit categories. If you don't fit every definition that's good for each form, most likely, no one would fit any of these characteristics. They're just to give you a sense of which one can relate and interact with you and better define you. You may feel that one reflects more of you than the other. Your intuitive style is important because it shows you how it affects your use of your psychic skills and the aspects, techniques, and abilities can come to you more naturally.

CHAPTER 21:

THE WORLD OF PROFESSIONAL PSYCHICS

The attitude of society towards psychics has shifted considerably throughout history, and I have certainly seen a great shift in the last thirty-five years. We do not need to meet in secret anymore. We are not on the stake charred. The representation of psychically talented people by Hollywood has changed and become more rational. I can rent a space to teach my psychic creation classes at our local community center and tell the landlord what the classes are about instead of making up some illusory words.

This is the good news that these gifts are certainly more accepted, but we still have a way to go. I always say to my students that breaking down myths is part of our role as psychics. Just like everybody has a certain psychic ability, so trained psychics are no different from everyone else.

Psychics are not just dark-haired, dark-eyed, scarf-wearing, earring hanging, black cat owners who read the minds of people, know when someone is going to die, and cheat people any chance they get, contrary to common belief. Hard-working, caring people are the majority of genuinely talented psychics I have encountered. Most have a sense of modesty regarding their gifts, and they know that the gifts come from God, so they take seriously the obligation that goes with these gifts. It's been my experience that at first, most genuinely talented psychics battle their abilities and go through a surrender process. Among all today's well-known psychics, not one of them grew up in the expectation of becoming a psychic.

To learn and develop and live their lives like anyone else, psychically talented people are here. We're dads and mothers, brothers and sisters, daughters and sons. We work hard, we fight bills, and we support our children with their homework. Most go to church or synagogue. We have interests and pets (and these are not just black cats!). We shop at the mall, bake cookies, mow the lawn, do volunteer work, and strive to grow like everyone else as human beings. In short, we are ordinary folks who are still learning about our talents and how to work with them.

Also, it is important to note that not all psychics are alike. Our gifts and abilities vary. People always believe that I will contact their deceased relatives, such as John Edward or James Van Praagh, but I can't do what they are doing. That's not how things work.

Psychics also specialize in a particular field. Some are very good at connecting (and are called 'mediums') with the deceased. Others are really good at finance and the stock market, like my brother Michael, and they do lectures that concentrate on business. Some concentrate on past lives, while others reflect on the future entirely. There are psychically talented individuals whose talent is to see health issues within a body (they are also referred to as "medical intuitives"). Some psychics can see and hear ghosts and support them (and call themselves "paranormal detectives" or "ghostbusters") on the other hand. Others can see and read the aura of a person, which is the field of energy surrounding our body. Certain psychics can accomplish many of these items, and others show their abilities in either one or two ways. My specialties are interacting with a person's spirit and helping individuals recognize their reasons for being here. I clearly see past lives. I can read sick bodies, and I can see and hear spirits and help them through to the other side.

When I was taking my psychic creation class, I recall our instructor telling us that we each have our own special way of communicating our gifts. She warned us not to compare in class with each other because it would discourage us only from discovering our own true gifts. She advised us to figure out what works best for us and reinforce that ability, which is what most of the experienced psychics I know have done.

STEREOTYPES

See the Sam Raimi film, *The Gift,* which stars Cate Blanchett, for an example of what life can still be like for a psychic today. The film accurately reflects the common doubts and perceptions that society has about genetically talented individuals, and it gives a good taste of how insane Christian fundamentalists can get. In the final court scene, Blanchett is cross-examined by the prosecuting attorney with stereotypical questions of what people think about psychics. Blanchett's response is, sadly, also typical of how defensive psychics often get.

Fortunately, as well-known psychics educate the public about themselves and their talents, this is changing. At the end of this book, I have included the first-hand, personal accounts of five psychically gifted individuals. They graciously agreed to answer a few questions and share a bit about themselves so you could gain a deeper understanding of psychics—lives, their talents, and their similarities and differences.

1-800 HOTLINES

For millions of people, the 1-800 paranormal hotlines on late-night TV are their only exposure to psychics. Miss Cleo was a favorite for late-night watchers, with her bright turbans and large hoop earrings, announcing the wonderful predictions she might make for our lives before she was busted for false ads.

Psychic hotlines have been a simple punchline for stand-up comedians for years, with the joke that the psychics who work the phones are all frauds. I had the chance to attend a private party for Dionne Warwick and some of the psychics working her hotline in 1994 at Planet Hollywood in Minneapolis. They were traveling from town to town to promote their show, and one of their stops was the Mall of America in Minneapolis. I brought my secretary with me, and both of us were happily shocked by the two psychics who were giving us lectures. They knew nothing about us, but we were sitting with Dionne at the head table. Robert from New York, the psychic who worked with me, said he wanted to read me because I was sitting with "the boss." He didn't ask for my name or anything else about me. He just stepped in and gave me some details about my job, book, finances, and love life. He was remarkably right, and the psychic who read her had the same experience with my assistant.

On her hotline, where all of the psychics just as good? I do not have a clue. Are all the psychics on late-night TV for real? I wish I could tell you that all the psychics you see on TV come from a position of honesty, and you can trust them, but I can't tell you that. Every profession has scam artists, and I have no idea what the ratio will be on these hotlines. I asked Robert why, rather than going out on his own, he wanted to work for the psychic network, and he said he didn't want the hassle of selling himself. He also said he liked the people who worked there, and being involved with it was a great business.

Shortly after the event for Dionne Warwick, I met a young woman working on another psychic network. She didn't know who I was or what I was doing for a living. I asked her how she got her psychic details, and she said that as she went along, she made things up. When I asked her if she had any psychic skills, she looked at me as if she had no idea what I was talking about and said, "Oh, whatever the bills were paying." I stood dumbfounded there. I didn't bother to send her my talk about honesty and integrity among psychics because she couldn't care less obviously. I discovered shortly after this experience that the woman was no longer working on the hotline, and I was relieved to hear it.

I hate it when people may not come from a position of honesty in my career, but it's not reasonable to believe that everyone would. Any career includes scam artists. In possessing psychic powers, there is nothing intrinsic that makes people act honestly or dishonestly. But again, as in every profession, with a bad rap, a few high-profile frauds can potentially taint all the psychics.

HOW TO SPOT SCAM ARTISTS

The first thing to bear in mind is that scam artists are in it for the money, no matter their supposed occupation. Many years ago, at a concert, someone came up to my dad and told him that she could see dark clouds in his aura, which meant that he was in danger ahead of him, but for a mere five thousand dollars, this horrible curse could be cleared and shielded from harm. Fortunately, my dad declined, but he called me as soon as he got home to ask if it was possible to do anything like this. It was complete garbage, I told him, and not to give it another thought. However, many people out there don't know who to call or message via one of these so-called psychics when they receive "bad news."

A woman sent me four separate letters she had received in the mail from different individuals claiming to be psychics while I was working on this segment. Each letter predicted some sort of doom and gloom and asked for a fee to help the writer get rid of this bad thing that was happening in her life. One letter spoke of a curse laid on her: "This is your last chance. The curse has to be broken within the next twenty-four hours, and your miracles have to begin.

Another letter said she was the "psychic illusion" of this woman and in the illusion of the woman they had met the previous night. The letter went on and on about different negative symbols in the woman's dreams and what she had to do to fend off this negativity, which included giving the psychic dream twenty-five dollars to perform the "Archangel Gabriel's Dream Rite." Another four-page letter went on warning this woman about the negative things that would happen to her on particular dates if she did not give her. Equally pathetic was the last message, except that this psychic wanted to double the amount, fifty dollars, to eliminate "the black cloud that surrounds its aura."

These prices could sound small, but believe me, they're just the beginning. Until these scam artists know they've got somebody scared of black clouds, or curses, or whatever, they're going to keep demanding more and more money. I've heard tales of people who ultimately paid so-called psychics thousands of dollars to shield them from evil events. Whenever and wherever they arise, these cases are all so profoundly tragic, but they have little to do with real psychic gifts. Scam artists will always try and intimidate you and then say that they are the only ones who can help and for a fee. These are the individuals to look out for.

If you're looking for a psychic right now, here are some very easy tips:

- If necessary, just go to someone to whom a good friend has referred you.

- Check your instincts if you are thinking about going to a psychic, or interviewing one: Is this the right time for you to do it? Is this the right one? Trust in the answer.

- If you're going through a traumatic, fragile period—like losing a loved one by death or divorce, finding out you're having a serious health problem, losing your job, finding out your child is on drugs, and so on—don't run to the first psychic you may find. It is normal to want to know how those things will work out when times are difficult, but when we feel desperate, we are vulnerable too, and that's what scam artists count on. Give yourself time to relax your nerves when you feel panicked, and then inquire around for a reliable psychic who can help you get through the situation. Twice you don't have to be victimized.

IDENTIFYING WHO IS WHO

In the Bible, Matthew 7:15-20, there is an excellent section on how to distinguish between a false prophet and the real deal that I believe applies to all professions: "Beware of false prophets who are dressed as harmless sheep but are actually wolves who will tear you apart. By how they behave, you can detect them, just like you can identify a tree by its fruit. You don't pick thornbushes for grapes or thistles for figs. A healthy tree generates good fruit, and poor fruit produces an unhealthy tree. A good tree can not produce bad fruit, and a bad tree can not produce good fruit. So any tree that doesn't yield good fruit is cut down and thrown into the flames. Yes, the way a tree or an individual can be defined is by the kind of fruit made.

If a person with psychic abilities is decent and honest and comes from a position of honesty, they will not have to advertise. Word of mouth will spread, and the person will have all the work they can manage. The person will yield fine fruit. If a person is not mentally talented but claims to be, they will not yield good fruit, and their company will not thrive. It is just as plain as this.

MISCONCEPTIONS ABOUT PSYCHICS AND THEIR ABILITIES

A friend of mine stayed at a Chicago hotel during Happy Hour that gave psychic readings, so she figured she might try it out. When she sat down, the psychic asked her whether she wanted to examine her handwriting, read a card (using a normal card deck), or read her palm. One of the most common misconceptions regarding psychics is that these kinds of "readings" are characteristic of psychics, but please note that none of these methods directly connects with true psychic gifts.

Even within my field, there can be uncertainty about the word "psychic." I've consulted with psychics over the past thirty-five years, attended conferences and psychic fairs, educated psychic people, and went to several psychics to see how others work. I've found that not everyone who claims to be a psychic is psychically gifted. When offering a reading, true psychics are people who use clairvoyance, clairaudience, and/or clarification. Tarot or otherwise, they don't need cards. They don't have to know your date of birth (that is astrology). They needn't read rune stones or the I Ching. They don't need your handwriting for a study. They don't need to look at your palm or consult an Ouija board. A true psychic does not need other resources than the gifts given to him by Nature. While some skilled psychics may use these techniques to assist, they rely mainly on their abilities.

Many people who have not mastered their psychic skills, unless they have trained to use these techniques, would call themselves "psychics." They depend entirely on these resources for information. However, I like to name these people fortune-tellers and not dismissively because they tell the future based on the cards, stones, or board. On the first night of class, I always advise my students that if they want to use any of these resources, they wait until they have completed the course and developed their skills first. Then they can use any of these supports in their job if they want to.

Indeed, it is not always easy to perceive psychic knowledge, and these resources will help explain the messages we receive. Let's say, for instance, a man goes to a clairvoyant to figure out why he hasn't met Ms. Right, and the clairvoyant gets an image of a cave in her third eye. Her task is to interpret the meaning of that picture correctly. She will enlist her intuition if she has learned how to work through her gift of sight and consider different interpretations to see which one gets a positive answer. Maybe she is asking her intuition, does the cave symbolize an insociable individual? Just kind of. Loner? Coming near. Not much contact with the world outside? Quick there. Is this person shy? Most of the time, he stays home and doesn't make himself available to the opposite sex? Bingo!-Bingo! That's the right reply.

When the clairvoyant gets the right meaning, the intuition will offer a firm nudge of yes.

Now, let's presume the same person asks the tarot card reader why he didn't meet Ms. Right, and in this particular case, the tarot card reader would possibly draw the Hermit card. With different tarot decks, this card's meaning varies, but the basic interpretation is that the person spends a lot of time in seclusion. When reading the pictures in a general way, the cards may be helpful, but if the reader is not psychic, then the cards' responses will be minimal.

MISCONCEPTIONS

It was fast approaching the end of the year, and I received a call from a reporter who said he was writing an article called "Having a Psychic Reading for the New Year." He needed some general data, such as prices and what people might expect for their money. The subject of his post, which introduced this as a fun idea, and asked him if he had ever been to a psychic for a reading, took me a little aback. He hadn't, so I clarified that getting a new year reading might not always be a pleasant experience as there are so many things that might go on in a person's life, both good and bad, and you might not want to hear about them all. In reality, years ago, on New Year's Eve, a friend of mine asked me if I would take a psychic to peek at what was in store for him next year.

The first sight that came to me was of some dark clouds. Then I saw his sister with both legs cast in the hospital, his brother trapped in a wheelchair, his mother getting a stroke, and my friend attending a funeral for someone. He will spend much of the year taking care of other people, my guides said. I remember wishing he hadn't asked me to read it, and I was trying to give him the details as politely as I could so that it wouldn't confuse him. Surely this experience was a good lesson for both of us not to look at psychic readings as a form of entertainment.

I bumped into my friend at the funeral of one of our mutual friends several months after the reading and he told me that all four predictions had come true. He said he wished he hadn't asked when I first gave him the details, but looking back, he was glad he was mentally prepared for everything as it happened.

The reporter and I ended up spending nearly an hour talking about psychics on the phone and the false claims that people make about us. People with psychic experience often cling to these myths, perpetuated by movies, horror stories, religion, and common culture. Here is a list of most common misconceptions:

We Are Constantly Emotionally Tuned Into People and World Affairs

This is a fallacy as far as being turned into world affairs twenty-four hours a day, seven days a week. Psychics don't know what's happening seven days a week, twenty-four hours a day. This is not to suggest that there are some things we don't experience. Many psychics may feel the approach of natural disasters, and many psychics thought that something terrible would happen around the date of the U.S. 9/11 terrorist attacks.

To my understanding, though, no psychics were able to pinpoint what would happen exactly or when. In any case, regularly tuning into world affairs will be such an energy drain that I can't imagine doing it.

Most experienced psychics that I know shield themselves from feeling these occurrences because there's nothing we can do about them anyway, as we've learned the hard way. Many of the trained psychics, just like anyone else, take a break from their jobs. Most of us make sure that our talents are "turned off" to not gather information from or about people when we're out of the public.

Psychics Read the Minds of Humans

This is such a fascinating one because we can't read people's minds knowingly; on the one hand, the answer is no. This is a fascinating issue, though, because psychics who are blessed with clairaudience, what we call mental telepathy, sometimes unknowingly pick up thoughts from other people. It has been my experience that when I pick up on someone around me's thoughts, I usually don't realize they're the thoughts of someone else. I have only recently begun consciously experimenting with mental telepathy to see if, in my own mind, I can tell the difference between my random thoughts and the thoughts of other people around me. I am slowly learning how to distinguish between the two, although this is not easy. Will we be consciously reading the minds of people? No. Should we take their feelings to heart? Yeah.

Psychics See Deep, Dark Secrets of People

This response is comparable to the last. We can't see people's secrets purposely, but if a person thinks very hard about a secret that they're hoping we can't see, a psychic can pick it up simply because the thoughts are out there. Another way to look at this is that we don't pick up people's deep dark secrets at random unless they ask us to.

Psychics Will Instinctively Know When People Will Die, and How

"This is one of those questions," I wish I had a dollar for each time anyone asked me. The reply, plain and simple, is no. The information about how or when a person will die is not open to psychics because it is not possible to predict. The few times I saw someone's death before it happened, the information was given to me by the person's soul with strict orders not to share the information with the individual.

Psychics Will See Future fot Themselves

Whenever something out of the ordinary happens in my life, someone normally asks me how come I didn't know it would happen, but one of the ironic facts about being psychic is that you are the hardest person to interpret. Although a psychic can predict his or her future, it is difficult because you need to be emotionally disconnected from all of the knowledge to interpret the information you receive accurately. This may sound simple, but it's virtually difficult to stay distant when it comes to your own life. The even greater irony is that he or she can see a lot about his or her life and future once a psychic (or anyone, for that matter) reaches that degree of emotional detachment. Still, once you've been that distant, you've reached the point where you generally don't care what's coming. Your mindset is clear that, if it comes, you take the good with the bad.

Psychics who seek psychic knowledge about their own lives generally go to other psychics or obtain their knowledge in meditation if they can isolate emotionally.

Psychics Know the Numbers for the Winning Lottery

Again, this is one of those times where we need to be fully disconnected to get specific lottery numbers because typically, when you're playing the lottery, you're playing to win. You're not emotionally disconnected from it.

Psychics Are All on a Spiritual Path

That's a misunderstanding I've had for years now. Since psychic gifts come from God and that being on a spiritual path is significant, I thought that all psychics believed this. However, I have encountered a few psychically gifted individuals since then who do not share my values or pursue a spiritual course. We are as diverse as people anywhere, and our values have little to do with our talents than with the values with which we have been educated, our life experiences, and the degree to which our soul has advanced.

All Psychics Function Alike

In terms of how we function, we are similar, but we each have our own way of communicating our abilities.

Every Psychic Reads Palms

Reading palms isn't an automatic aspect of the psychic being. They have taken a class or learned it from a book if someone reads the palms.

Psychics See Only Positive Things

If that were only real, it would make my job so much easier, but it is not. As my friend figured out when he asked for that New Year's Eve reading, we see the good and the negative.

Psychics Know Where All the Missing Kids Are

It's a heartbreaker, this one. I sure wish we could trace all the missing kids, pets, and adults—as well as their captors—but that can be really hard to do. It is literally like finding a needle in a haystack. As I explained earlier, psychic knowledge does not arrive like a telegram with all of the specifics spelled out. Psychics may see or feel whether a person is dead or alive. They can get photos of wooded areas or water bodies, but precisely pinpointing an exact position is very difficult. Furthermore, the more the psychic is emotionally involved, the more complicated it would be, as the psychic may block relevant details because they do not want to see the truth of the situation.

The Same Is True of Psychic Abilities and Intuition

Not the same things are psychic abilities and intuition, and those two positions are different. Clairvoyance and clairaudience are located in our head; clairsentience is a body sensation. Depending on the individual, intuition is our inner awareness located in our solar plexus, heart, or gut region.

Psychic Abilities Are Evil

It can only be bad motives, not psychic powers themselves. Our other five senses are similar to psychic abilities: they are a way of obtaining knowledge. It is up to us to what we do with that knowledge. This question is most frequently posed by devoutely religious people, and in subsequent chapters, I answer what the Bible has to say about psychic ability.

Psychic Interpretations Are Written In Stone

Remember often that the psychics can misunderstand the information they get, and the prediction's timing may be off. Using your own instincts, it is also necessary to determine any psychic reading, which will let you know whether the information is correct or not. Psychic forecasts; however, don't eradicate free will; the decisions will make a difference. Only because a prediction is made by a psychic does not mean that it will come true.

Psychics Can Obtain Very Specific Details

I can not tell you the number of women who asked if I could give them their husbands 'mistress' name, address, and telephone number. We don't receive this kind of information.

We get general knowledge that is unique, as confusing as this sounds. We can get a physical description, a first name, and the town in which the woman lives, but not the minute specifics people assume we can (like the particular cave in which Bin Laden is hiding).

The Psychics on TV Represent All Psychics

Nowadays, people immediately think of the high-profile ones on TV, like James Van Praagh on Beyond, John Edward on Crossing Over, or Sylvia Browne, when someone mentions the word psychic. People believe that all psychics are just like the ones on TV, but it's just not like that. We are as diverse as any other group of random people. By making entertaining shows, TV producers make a living. Besides choosing precise and fast psychics, they want those who are also beautiful, polished, humorous, pleasant, and not overwhelmed through cameras or crowds. Most of the psychics I know are simply introverts—they'd rather get a root canal than do their work in front of cameras, knowing millions are watching. In the privacy of their home or workplace, most psychics tend to read their customers because they know the data that comes through is also very personal. Since producers dislike dead-air time or feel that they have to "perform," they just want to do their job without any strict time limits.

A thick skin is one attribute that I think is necessary for TV psychics to have. You become a victim of debunkers and those who have little regard for the profession by being a public personality. Most psychics I know are very sensitive and would not be ready for criticism to become a lightning rod. Ultimately, I would say that it is rare for an individual to have all the qualities necessary to be effective on a television show.

CHAPTER 22:

HOW TO IMPROVE YOUR MENTAL HEALTH

Now that we've been through the four styles of psychic messaging and you've realized that you're better with one than the other, as well as having discovered your intuitive form, let's talk about how to practice and reinforce those abilities.

Get off to the road to feeling motivated and positive in yourself! Remember, even the most skilled or naturally talented psychics did not begin their journey with full trust and power; they also had to work to increase their skills gradually. The trick is to remain calm and believe in yourself. Trust in your ability and instincts, even though it can seem naive at first if you've been raised to deny it. Continue to note little things you feel. Besides, bear in mind that, as longer sessions are overly taxing and exhausting, you should bear practice sessions reasonably short, no more than an hour, as you can't be expected to keep your attention that long. Any exercise you attempt will be unsuccessful once you have lost your concentration and grounding.

When you start to have more accurate premonitions, a feeling of fear can arise. This is inevitable—you are now conscious of a plane of life with which human beings are not usually in harmony. Part of building your skills and trust is to resolve this apprehension or uneasiness. If you just want to become better, then fear can just get in the way. Reluctance will hamper you. It is true that not every forecast is going to be a good one. You can predict relationships that end or lose money or death, and you have to understand that both of these are a part of life. Also, you have to be prepared for unpleasant premonitions.

Another important thing to note is: don't let skeptics deter you from doing so. You would know if you have had a psychic experience that, while rationality can not justify it, there is no denying its validity. They might ridicule you or challenge you if there are many hardcore logical skeptics in your life, trying to persuade you that you're dumb or even insane. Staying calm and concentrated is essential; don't let these kinds of people distract you or hinder your skills. Everywhere you are going to find people like them, so try to block them out as best you can.

Writing down possible psychic messages is one excellent strategy. Try to maintain a record of what you believe might be premonitions that are clairvoyant, sensory, sentient, or conscious. Keep track of these videos, and see if anything ever becomes important to them—if at all. For beginners, this is an ideal method because you can pick out the random bits and pieces from real psychic signals, and you can start piecing together what a prediction or premonition feels like. It can also help you write down how you feel next to each possible post.

This can not be adequately repeated. Day-to-day activity. This could sound overwhelming, but if you keep it up, it'll come easily pretty quickly, and you won't even know that you're doing it. Now, if for whatever reason you miss a day or two or more (illness, feeling emotionally exhausted, etc.), don't worry! Only pick up where you left off and keep checking various methods and instruments. If you haven't exercised in a while, it's not anything to worry over; you won't lose "the talent" as we all have it, just as if you don't go to the gym for a while, the muscles won't deteriorate. This is just to inform you of the best and most successful ways of developing the power of your gift.

Meditation is another highly powerful instrument. In subsequent chapters, we will go over it more extensively, but we will now touch on it as it is one of the key instruments and strategies for improving your psychic intuition.

If you are regularly practicing, before you try to interpret something, try integrating ten to twenty-minute meditation sessions into your daily routine. This will clear any emotional blockages, feelings, fears, or distractions that might be important to your psychic practice or to your everyday life. It also ties you to a higher dimension where the guide(s) of your spirit and psychic energies reside. Connecting during meditation with your spirit guide(s) would also help answer any questions you may have, as they will help you. Meditation empties your mind to better concentrate your attention on the spiritual mission at hand. See Chapter 25 for more detail about meditation, meditation methods, and spirit guides.

Also, psychometry is a very simple technique to try. The word may sound complicated, but it's all about reading an object's energy. Just pick up something you know has some value, like a family heirloom to begin with, and concentrate on the energy that comes out of it. Clear your mind and see what happens. Do not force images to flow; only let them flow. Try switching to an item you do not know the past and significance of until you have practiced like this a few times. Go to a thrift shop and buy an old silver knick-knack or jewelry piece. Or you can ask a friend to give you their or their family's valuable things without telling you about the past and significance behind them. This way, it is likely to be more productive as you can read in front of your friend, tell them what pictures, words, or feelings are coming up, and they can tell you whether they are important or correct.

Notice certain images reoccurring in your premonitions. If you've done some preliminary research on prophecies or forecasts, you'll probably have come across some kind of symbol guide—stuff like red means passion, 13 means bad luck, green means richness, etc. What you need to remember; however, is that there are no universals! For everyone, symbols are different. The idea of trying to keep tabs on what specific pictures, colors, or numbers seem to symbolize to you is connected to the journal idea.

If possible, surround yourself with people of the same mind as you, such as other psychics or people following the same spiritual path. If you find others at the same vibration level, the energy will increase, which will help you spiritually flourish. Increase your psychic ability, then. It's also good for your peers to provide positive reinforcement. Try finding any online if you don't know someone in your life with a similar concept of spirituality. Different social media groups or forums may be just as useful as advice and discuss face-to-face. If you can enter and participate in any local groups where you live, you can even lookup. Try searching for a combination of seasoned psychics and inexperienced psychics. That way, you can get advice from the more seasoned members and ask questions while not feeling too intimidated as you have other beginners to practice and compare notes with. It's essential to have positive support from like-minded people, whether online or in your life.

It's also a stress reliever to spend time in nature to help expand your mind. Some of this may just sound like simple life advice that doesn't have anything to do with psychic powers. Still, if you are depressed and emotionally / energetically blocked, it's impossible to progress as a psychic. Nature has its origins in us. Before us, nature was here, and it will stay here even after we pass by. Walk around and remember that the trees will still stand firm, amid all your concerns. Even the wind will whistle. You're not going to avoid the world. Take in nature's peace and ancient energies and let those energies soothe the mind and clear it. An empty mind is the best way to start a psychic reading, as mentioned.

Ask frequently asked questions about the Universe. Whether you're walking down the sidewalk and wondering if you ought to change careers, or whether you're relaxing in the bath, wondering if your relationship works out? Try to become aware of this and consciously ask the universe for advice, no matter where you are and what you are wondering about. Take it out of the wondering state, and ask the universe purposefully, what am I doing? How do I grasp this? Just get specific. You might not get an immediate reply, but if you wait a day, a week, maybe a couple of weeks, the reply will likely be sent to you. You just need to ask.

If these techniques have been tried and you feel like you're stuck on what to do next, just repeat, repeat, repeat, practice, practice, and practice. For everyone, the path to developing your psychic powers is different, but staying confident and focused is the universal one. If there's one method that seems like it works better for you than the others, concentrate on the one—everything that works best to improve your forces.

Next, we will cover some important instruments that psychics often use: tarot, scrying crystal ball, palmistry, and reading tea leaf. Both these are ways of divination, a way to say the future. Psychics can use other physical instruments and techniques, but let's start with those four. You would probably choose one over the others or find that a certain technique comes much more easily and is simpler for you, giving you more precise readings. Do not feel pressure to learn them all; they are only potential tools you can use as psychics.

If you've ever heard of tarot cards, you've probably heard that you can't buy your own deck; you've got to have one. It's a myth here. You can select and buy your own deck, and nothing can change that. Try to communicate with it when selecting a deck. The energy has to interact with you. This is also a good sign that it's your deck if the artwork really stands out to you. Don't try and do some readings right away once you've picked your deck. You have to "break it in" emotionally. One way to do this is to take each card out one-by-one and smoke it over. This will purify its energy. Then shuffle through the deck and examine each card, taking in any emotions that may evoke the artwork. Go to your deck for a walk, and sleep with it next to your pillow. It's important that your energies are intertwined so that the deck is familiar with you.

You can do the readings for yourself when you're just starting, and then perhaps ask a friend if you can practice with them. You can find a spread you like when you do a reading (for example, three cards: one for the past, one for the present, and one for the future) and ask the card a question while shuffling / before spreading them out. It can not be a yes or no question because there are no cards or yes. It can be as ambiguous or descriptive as you want. However, they may want to keep their question private if you do a reading for someone else, but let them know that this may make it slightly harder to interpret the cards' meaning. If you're reading for someone else, lay the deck in front of them and ask them to break the deck into three piles, then pick the top card from each pile (this is one example of a simple spread. If there's another way you like you want them to draw the cards, or if you want to draw for them, then go for it, there are a lot of different techniques). Check to see if all of them are upside-down when each card is flipped over, showing the artwork (decide first which way will be the right way up, face you, or face them). Not everybody now holds that assumption, but many tarot readers read upside-down cards differently than when they were up the right way.

This way, you can read or disregard them. Your tarot pack was supposed to come with a small book explaining every card. If not, then you can go out and purchase a tarot book or check online from your nearest occult shop or bookstore. However, the definition is just half that. The next step is to apply it to the person's question/life and translate it according to what they have asked. If they don't want to answer your question, explain the meanings of the cards and where they sit as best you can in the spread, and consult with them to see if it makes sense and relates to their question at all. Some readings would be highly apparent in their post, while others are more cryptic and require more study and introspection. Get into the habit of drawing one card every morning to see how your day will go to practice memorizing card meanings and explanations. Choose your card and read the summary therefor. You will become more acquainted with the cards and their details pretty quickly.

Crystal scrying ball is another classic technique psychics use. It's such a common thing that it's found its way into many movies, and it's a universal psychic icon. Although it is such a popular icon, it is an art that is difficult to perfect and most probably will not achieve immediate or solid results. To get started, it is best to yell crystal ball in a dimly lit ambient space that allows the mind to relax and wander. Large balls of the crystal can be pretty costly, but tiny ones work just as well and cheaper. Make sure it's a transparent ball of crystal and not made of an opaque stone, and that you have some kind of stand for it (it's preferable to plastic to wood, glass, or stone) so that it doesn't just fall off the table. You should concentrate on the middle while you look into your crystal ball.

Try to have some kind of solid background behind you, so as not to distort the image, as some objects or light can be mistaken for images. You can feel like you are entering an almost trancelike state, and it may take a couple of minutes for the ball to start revealing stuff to you. Note, the secret is relaxation. Light incense or diffuse essential oils, and play soothing ambient music if you think this will help you get to the right state where the mysteries of the ball will show itself. Before you begin, take a moment to quiet your mind. Clear it of any hopes or dreams of what you believe will happen or what you believe you are going to see. Before you start, another thing to remember is spending time getting acquainted with your crystal ball, like with your tarot deck.

Keep it close to you, create the connection. You can start looking now that you're ready, your mind relaxed, your mood set. Make sure that for an extended period, whatever place you sit into gaze will be relaxed, as it can take a while for messages to be shown, or if it's your first time, not at all, and you'll have to stay in one place for a while to keep your attention. When you look, envision that your mind is as pure as a ball of crystal. When a mist starts emerging, you'll know a message is coming in. Do not move, either physically or mentally, as this occurs. Try staying focused and maintaining the connection. Keep cool and quiet. You can be drawn into the crystal ball and your mind, the ball, and you are one. Images will surface, but they will not be interpreted yet. Only take them in, ingest them as they appear, all one-by-one, until they begin to fade. This is when you're able to break your concentration.

You will now look back upon all that you have seen. View the images as you would a letter or a dream of clairvoyance. What did they symbolize? What were they trying to tell you about someone or some issue in your life (or the person you're reading for)? How has that been represented? If you keep a journal of your psychic activities and experiences, write down any vision that showed itself to you during your gaze on your crystal ball in as much detail as possible so you don't forget. Then you can go back to them later and examine it. Know, you can not see anything the first time or for the first few times. Crystal ball scrying is a very difficult technique to learn and hone, so just keep trying not to get frustrated and do your best.

Another popular symbol of psychic practice is palmistry (or chirology), and another helpful method many psychics use to perform readings. Mastering it is much simpler than scrying a crystal ball and cheaper than purchasing a crystal ball or tarot box. All you need is a person who is willing to let you hold their hands for a short period of time, and that doesn't cost any money at all. Your nearest psychic shop may have been decorated with a neon sign of a hand with all the lines used by palm readers to tell you about your life. A line reflects something about a different person. There's the line of life, the half-circle that begins from the center of your hand and curves around your thumb.

The line of head and the line of heart running parallel to each other (the head is the lower line, the line of heart higher, closer to the fingers). There's also the line of fate that slices through the heart and headline, but not everybody has a line of fate. These are only a couple of the most fundamental lines you can interpret on somebody's side. Health, illness, significant life events, and wellness are reflected in the life line. The head line reflects how someone thinks and interacts, how someone is imaginative or intelligent, and how someone learns. The line of heart stands for feeling, romance, relationships, mental wellbeing, and heart health. The line of fate reveals how much of someone's life is governed by "destiny" or forces beyond their control.

Look at your own hand to see if you can pinpoint each line. How you read them is dependent on how the line on the hand appears. Longer and more curvy lines mean more emotional and imaginative, while lines that are straight and shorter display a strong handle on emotions and a rational disposition. Line breaks, particularly the lines of life and destiny, signify major life changes. There are several online books and blogs where you can read about how different lines tend to mean different things, but here are some examples of this:

- Life Line: the closer your life line is to your thumb, the tireder and the less stamina you seem to have. The stronger and longer a life-line is, the more liveliness someone has. The shorter and shallower the person is, the weaker the will. If your life line is straight and does not bend much towards the base of the thumb, when it comes to romance, you are probably careful. A circle or island in the line of your life can mean injury.

- Head Line: the person has more physical capacity than mental capacity if it's short. There's a love of adventure present if it's isolated from the line of life. A curved head line shows the person being imaginative. A wavy head line shows a brief period of focus. If the line is long and wide, then the person is a simple, logical thinker. If it's a straight line, then they're a realist. This may be a sign of emotional trauma if someone has a circle or cross in their head line. Scattered thought may be reflective of a split headline.

- Heartline: if the heart line stops below the index finger (or begins depending on how you read it), the person will be content with his love life. If it stops under the middle finger, then the person is selfish when it comes to love and romance. If it stops in the center of the hand, then the person is likely to have no trouble falling in love. If the line is really short and straight, then the subject is not involved in romance. If the line of heart crosses the line of life, has smaller lines crossing it, or is broken up, both of these may be indicators of heartbreak. This can show depression or a time of grief if there's a circle or island inside it. If it is a long and curvy line, the person is emotional, but if it is quite straight and runs very parallel to the title, they can easily regulate their emotions. If it's a wavy line, they most likely have trouble with commitment and have probably had many romantic partners.

- Fate Line: the deeper the line, the more the individual is influenced by "fate" and/or external powers, the more the individual has the power of his or her own life. If there are many breaks in the line of destiny, with many variations, it demonstrates life. This shows someone who has many potentials and is self-made when it's joined with the lifeline at the bottom. If it joins the middle of the lifeline, this indicates a person who has or will be setting aside their interests for someone else's. If it goes through the lifeline, this person will have a wide network of support throughout their lives.

There's also a distinction in which hand you're reading. Your dominant hand will be your hand, past and present, showing everything that a person has been born with. Anything that will happen in your future will be revealed by your non-dominant side. So, whatever you see on their dominant hand is something that has already happened and tells you about it, while whatever is exposed to their non-dominant hand is the stuff that could still become. Reading both hands is better for getting the full picture and giving the individual the best reading you can give.

However, these forecasts are not set in stone, and there may be signs in someone's hand that show the power to alter what the future will bring, such as the line of destiny. Often, hand size counts. It is generally possible to identify someone with smaller hands as a doer, whereas someone with larger hands is more cerebral and takes less action. By balling up your fist, you can also discover how many children a person would have. Turn it around so you can see the folds that your pinky is creating. The number of free lines (not connecting the pinky with the palm) is the number of kids you'll get. However, this doesn't work for adopted kids.

The reading of Tea Leaf is focused on symbolism and what the psychic interprets in the images which the tea leaves produce. Coffee grounds may do this too, but tea leaves are the most popular way to use them. For this, you'll have to pour yourself a cup of loose-leaf tea. Obviously, a tea bag is not going to work. Drink the cup of tea you made. It's ok if there's a tiny bit of liquid at the bottom, as this will help with the next stage, which is keeping the cup in your hand for a moment, asking it a question (no yes or no questions), and spinning the now empty cup (save the tea leaves) in the opposite direction, three times. Now turn the cup upside down and leave for a moment so any extra liquid can slip away. Switch it on again on the right side and take a look at what you see.

Keep in mind something that jumps out at you instantly, or any sense that you get from your first look. If nothing leaps at you and everything seems really complicated and makes no sense, that's good too. Don't let it deter you. To see if something changes or looks different, you should look at the cup from different angles. Take your time, and slowly and thoughtfully, study all the shapes and clusters. Keep your mind open and relaxed when reading and concentrating on how the things you see could be relevant to the question you have asked. Try not to put a message on. Crosses, stars, letters or numbers, anchors, or natural formations, such as trees or flowers, are common symbols you might see. There is no universal way these symbols can be interpreted, but below is a list of some of the most common symbols and possible interpretations or meanings:

- **Ladder** – Erfolg. Typically in your life at work, but that may be any part of your life. You're "climbing" the ladder to achievement and success.

- **Gun** – This shows the will to act. Everything makes you upset and angry in your life, and you want to do everything about it.

- **Snake** – Hard times forecast to come. Probably to do with your work, maybe on the horizon, a life change. Brace for challenges yourself.

- **Mountains** – Mountains are typically a journey you have to follow or challenges you have to tackle on the way to the destination.

- **Angel** – This is a symbol of your spiritual side being in touch. You may enter a time of spiritual change and peace of mind.

- **Baby** – This symbol is positive. The interpretation of rebirth is an obvious one, as well as a life change and positive news. It could also be telling you a new opportunity could soon be yours.

- **Acorn** – The acorn is another common symbol seen in tea leaf reading. It is a sign that your hard work will be rewarded and that good news and opportunity are on their way to you.

- **Plane** – This symbol tells you to break out of stagnation in your life if you wish for success. There may also be an unexpected journey or a time-sensitive decision ahead of you.

- **Anchor** – A positive sign is an anchor. This shows that the relationships in your life are solid, and the people in your life are faithful, whether they are friendships, romantic commitments, or family ties. There is plenty of love there. It could be a hint too, that your dream will come to life.

- **Bird(s)** – Seeing birds in the tea leaves is another encouraging indication that good news is generally on its way. It's a premonition of coming positives. It also facilitates the making of choices.

- **Fish** – Seeing fish will mean good luck if something/someone comes to you or you fly overseas, or something to do with overseas.

- **Flowers** – Another fortunate omen. If there are several of them or love, flowers can also symbolize near platonic friendships.

- **Heart** – Happiness is entering your life. This may be because of someone you have affections for (they don't necessarily need to be romantic) or because they come in money. Or probably both! You'll be able to dream, right?

- **Cat** – The picture of a cat may mean that your life might be present with treachery, betrayal, gossip, or unkindness or unpleasantness. This may also mean differences with family or issues involving money.

- **Dog** – You might be struggling in everything you were trying to do. A picture of a dog may also foresee an unhappy end to a relationship, or again, money problems.

- **Triangle** – An unlikely but fruitful experience.

- **Tree(s)** – A symbol of happiness is a tree or plants. Money's coming your way; you're going to be prosperous. You are likely to be as content as you are safe and willing to.

Mind not to push the tea leaves on any photos you want to see. Naturally, let them appear to you—don't pretend to see something that isn't there or to distort the pictures to suit your fancy.

Also essential is the location of the tea leaves and where they end up in the cup. You (or the person who receives the tea leaf reading) are associated with tea leaves around the rim or handle, and most likely, they would be symbolic of the current or near future. Whatever is in the teacup bowl reflects things that are going to happen in the farther future. Another meaning is that the closer the handle is, the more the message is optimistic. Thus in the bowl, the farther down, the bad news this is. And generally, if it's in the cup, it can mean that this happens to someone in their life, a relative, mate, lover, or even acquaintance, not to the topic of the reading.

If you get frustrated and feel like you're not progressing or changing, don't forget to look back to see how far you've come! You're likely to feel better seeing the progress you've made and how much more you're in tune with your instincts. You may have honed in on your intuitive form, or you may have had a premonition that turned out real. Do not be compared to anyone! If they are more experienced than you or beginners like you who seem to make more progress, remember: the path is different and special to all! Reflect on your success and your own direction.

CHAPTER 23:

PSYCHIC PROTECTION

It is necessary to understand the possible risks involved and how to protect yourself from them, now that you are dabbling in the domain of psychic messaging and the spirit world. You are energetically and spiritually opening up and are vulnerable to harmful energies. Much like in the physical world, you want to protect yourself from these forces in the spiritual realm, just as you would avoid and protect yourself from negative and nasty individuals, locations, artefacts, etc., and the first step to protecting and curing yourself of psychic attack is to recognize what a psychic attack looks like.

Psychic assault is when someone sends negative energies or "spirits" to latch you on, intended dangerously and maliciously. Maybe they didn't really mean to or know they were doing it. They may not even be psychic or intuitive at all. Psychic attacks can be willed on you by someone who doesn't even believe in them; they can only hurl mighty destructive thoughts and curse your way. However, a paranormal attack isn't just coming from people. You must be precise about who or what kind of spirit you are asking when you meditate and invite spirits into your space or ask them for guidance, as if you leave your space open and leave your question general, some very dark "spirits" or forces may take advantage of this and enter your home, wreaking energetic havoc about your life and on your psychic abilities. This dark energy can throw away your psychic abilities, cause emotional suffering, and cause chaos in your life. Things just won't feel right when you're the victim of a psychic assault. This entity or spirit wants or wishes to harm you for some reason, and you need to know how to protect yourself in the event of a psychic attack.

How can you say whether you're the victim of a mental assault or just going through a rough patch in life? Nightmares, particularly very vivid nightmares, fear of a particular room in your home, feeling a presence/feeling of being watched, bad luck, sudden illness, depression, and/or fatigue, objects falling over in your home even though no one touched them, feeling like your energy has been drained, unable to focus your strength or feeling goosebumps. Please bear in mind that these are not promises that you were targeted for a psychic attack; many of the items on the list can be just a part of life, and this is not a complete list either. Nevertheless, keep an eye on whether some/all of these symptoms arise in your life, and whether those feelings are natural for you, or are obviously coming from nowhere. The odds are that if you have one or a lot of these, it's a psychic attack. If you're usually someone with nightmares and poor luck, then maybe there's no supernatural force behind it. If you're a paranoid individual that still feels like being monitored, then there's definitely no nefarious enemy behind these emotions. However, if all of these occur together, and it's particularly out of the ordinary, beginning to put up any psychic defenses wouldn't hurt.

Through imagination, the best and easiest way to repel negativity is, though, it takes a lot of energy. You can imagine this in a few different ways. One example is: just close your eyes and imagine that you are surrounded by radiating blinding white light (or a color of your choice that symbolizes strength and safety for you) if you feel negative presence or energies around you. Breathe in to harness the energy that fills you with this sun, and feel the strength to fill your body. As you exhale, imagine the light is shot out in a blinding burst to engulf everything in your radius, blasting any negativity well away from you, so that your whole vision is white for a moment. Inhale as the light disappears, and you are peacefully standing in the eye of your mind. To feel as if the negative presence has broken, repeat as many times as needed. To repel harmful powers, you can also create your own visualization. Just remember to channel a lot of energy into it;

otherwise, it isn't going to do anything better than a daydream would. Do not use your own energy, but tap into the energy of the world, so you do not exhaust yourself.

If you find that your psychic skills are becoming very powerful and you are being bombarded at all times by psychic "sixth sense" data, silk is a helpful tool to block the overload of knowledge. Try loosely carrying a silk scarf around your head, or draping over your shoulders and chest. Also, silk helps to protect the wearer from psychic attacks and prevent any attempted psychic attacks.

Incense is also a successful way to protect or cure psychological assault. The incense smoke cleanses the room and forces harmful energies out of it. Try to light the incense daily to keep your home safe. Or, if you think you are the victim of a psychic attack, light incense every day, particularly in any space, because of negative spirits/entities setting up camp there, you feel a unique sense of negativity, evil, or negative energy build-up. Keep on doing so until you sense the ebb of these destructive forces, and spiritually restore and cleanse you and your home. You may also meditate or sit in front of the incense to cleanse your mind and clear your mind, just make sure the ventilation is correct. Otherwise, the smoke will go straight to your lungs, and since there is nowhere for them to go, the negative entities will not be pushed out; they will remain in your room. This does not mean opening all the doors and windows if it's cold, just making a fan go in or slightly cracking a window before the incense goes out. Gemstones are another protection you can wear/carry with you. Certain gemstones have properties that repel negativity and supernatural attacks, such as the powerful black tourmaline or obsidian. Here is a list of some awesome gemstones for psychic attack avoidance and defense:

- **Tiger's eye**: tiger's eye is a heavy, effective stone for blocking other people's psychological attacks on you. It repels the evil eye and leaves helpless your assailant to hurt you.

- **Amethyst:** amethyst is kind of an all-purpose stone, but in this case, it is perfect for dissipating negative energy, especially negative energies that are directed at you. This turns them into something more meaningful.

- **Garnet:** fire is the feature of the gemstone garnet. This stone burns up and evaporates evil spirits and forces seeking to get into your house. It acts as an impressive shield.

- **Lapis Lazuli:** lazuli will enhance your trust and break down insecurity. It absorbs and then filters out the harmful spirits and energies, rendering them weak and harmless. You won't even know that they had ever been there.

- **Black Tourmaline:** black tourmaline is considered by many to be the greatest protective stone, especially against psychic attacks. For you, this is good news. It is a fast-acting stone that will neutralize any harmful energies or forces heading your way and break them up. They're not even going to make it anywhere near you.

- **Hematite:** like garnet, this stone can serve as a barrier against adverse presences and energies seeking to get at you. It is an extremely powerful shield, and it is also connected to the earth portion, making it good for grounding.

- **Labradorite:** a protection against psychological abuse as well as a defense against any harm or ill wished by another to you.

- **Black Obsidian:** this is a great stone. If you think you're being threatened by someone really wealthy, someone with a lot of psychological strength, you're uncertain if you can match. This is a perfect stone to blast their attempts at a psychic attack free, and a kind of bonus advantage is that bad luck is counteracted!

- **Peridot:** a great defensive stone against those that really drain your life. This stone is less for defense from an attack and more about when you're going to spend time with someone you know who has really negative energy and typically leaves you feeling very low in energy and exhausted afterward. Whether it's someone you care for, a friend who may be goes through depression, or a family member you think is dishonest and never has a positive word to say or a boss who does it. Whoever it is, you are shielded by this stone from its normal impact.

- **Quartz:** like amethyst, is another stone with very generic use. It dissolves and transforms negative energy.

- **Smokey Quartz:** smokey quartz is a very strong stone if you want to be more precise than clear quartz. It has a high defensive potential and also has healing properties. It also helps with anxiety, doubts, and struggles with self-esteem. It gives peace of mind and makes its wearer stronger.

- **Turquoise:** this stone is a stone for healing. Consider wearing turquoise on your patient if you are the victim of a psychological assault. It will shield you, and it will dissipate any harmful energy around you.

- **Salt:** salt is a helpful weapon to use as its energy-absorbing properties are useful when defending against harmful energies. Try to keep some salt around when calling on spirits in some way, whether you are doing mediumship, asking your spirit guides for advice, or welcoming a spirit into your room or speaking with spirits in general. You may sprinkle it around yourself or your room (a less messy way to do this is to absorb it in water and spray it around you or your space) and place a small pile in the four corners of your house or room sprinkle it over windowsills and doorsills.

Keep these stones on you, around you, or at all times in your home/space, and you will not even detect harmful presences, forces, or spirits that try to hurt you, and you will be blissfully unaware of any attempted (and thwarted) paranormal assault. Just remember: your stones absorb all these blows, so they'll need to be washed from time to time. This can be achieved by passing them over incense, leaving them out in the moonlight or sunlight (but sunlight can fade colorful crystals like amethyst, so don't use this strategy for those crystals), burying them in the soil for some time, or leaving them out in the rain (again, check to make sure that the crystals you leave in the rain or water are not water-soluble). You can also clean them energetically and draw all the built-up energies inside them, for more on how to do so. These are just some of the ways you can clean your crystals-choose what technique you want to use or what one seems more natural to you.

You may also hang mirrors from your walls or put mirror fragments in your lawn to mirror any planned damage to where it came from. You should ask for assistance from your spirit guides to protect yourself against attacks. Make sure you don't ask them for something—ask politely like you would ask a mentor for help. Know, your spirit guides monitor over you; they're on your side. If the attack is strong, you would need the additional help. If you have someone who also has psychic abilities in your life, trust them, they can give some helpful energy to battle the attack. The reflection surface of the mirrors should be facing outward, away from you. Both negative energies and spirits can be efficiently reflected away and bounce off the mirrors in this way.

Symbols and Sigils are excellent for protection as well. You may have heard people talk about your lucky horseshoe, your lucky underpants, or what you have. You may have heard people say, "Without my lucky item/symbol, I'm not going to go and do such a dangerous job." A symbol of security may be anything. Many people who practice pagan traditions use a pentagram for protection. This is the upward-facing 5-

pointed star, surrounded by a disk. There are significant signs of protection from many religions and cultures. Find a symbol, make your own, draw it, carve it, sew it, trace it onto something with your eye, or with a crystal or incense stick. The smart idea is to sew it into your pillow for defense against psychic attack, since that is where your head lies at night and your mind is, of course, going to be the object of psychic attack. When you have discovered your psychic sign, you have to make an energetic charge against it.

This means you'll want to concentrate on what you want this sigil to achieve and direct the sigil's energy and goal. Focus your attention and desire on this sigil when holding it in your lap, rubbing it, or tracing it with your finger over and over to physically express your attention and wish on it. What you want from the sign of security, its aim or intent, and what it should be doing, you can even talk out loud. This is yet another way of voicing your desire for it to energetically secure you. Get detailed about your assignment for it as well. Make sure that you want it to protect you from psychological attacks, that you are sick, any harmful forces, ghosts, beings, and people that wish you harm, and that your mind, body, soul, and energy are protected and that your well-being is assured. Of course, to speak to it, you should make your own chant or mantra, but these are just ideas for some things to add.

If you've already been the target of a psychological attack, recovering from it is the next move. In the paragraphs above, some strategies have been listed, but let's really get into what needs to be done to recover from a psychic attack, as the results can be very devastating.

After a paranormal attack, you'll probably feel very abused, so try to ground yourself. At a time like this, reflection, introspection, constructive thinking, and the encouragement of your loved ones would be important. Don't allow yourself out of control to spiral. Breathing exercises, along with meditation, will significantly help keep clear the psychic channels. Don't succumb to the dark energies sent to you. That's what will be desired by your attacker. If you know who the attacker is (or at least have a suspicion), you should imagine them with light and positive energy surrounding them. Sending this picture out into the world will help manifest the shutting down of this individual's destructive forces and weaken their will to do harm and send negativity out.

This method often extends to evil spirits and malicious beings if you consider the assailant to be supernatural in nature. If you have dreams, write them down and discuss them, it can make them seem less amazing and terrifying, and they can symbolize and represent issues, fears, and issues that need to be worked on in your waking life. If you experience an energy loss or sudden depression, trust someone and try and find the right ways to help improve the energy to function for you. Remember: this is a spiritual invasion, so concentrate on your soul, resources, and emotional well-being in your recovery.

You can feel stress and anxiety. It can be difficult to realize when you're right in it, but getting the understanding that these anxieties and panics aren't rooted in something logical can be calming. This is a symptom of a psychic attack, and half the fight is to identify signs. It does not stop the feeling to know that your anxiety, while it feels very real, is nothing to worry about. Still, ideally, there will be some small relief at the back of your mind knowing that it is not rooted in something real, no matter how uncomfortable it may feel when experiencing it.

Give one break to yourself. If necessary, take time off from all recovery and recuperation tasks. There is no point in coping with all the problems of life AND a psychic assault, which is simultaneously when you are at your lowest. This means taking a break from your psychic work! Consider it a sick day for the spiritual. Try not to get drawn into the mindset of the victims. Going down that path is so convenient, but then again, ground yourself. Remind yourself that you're strong. Find a visualization that works for you to inhale and exhale with your constructive power to repel the negative energies.

Wallowing in your symptoms to become a victim is playing into what your abuser wants. You are becoming weaker and more vulnerable to their assaults. If your symptoms become severe, of course, do not neglect them. Pay attention to yourself, but don't let you drown them. Find the power inside yourself, tap into the limitless energies of the world, build up, and heal yourself. Don't let worry reign over you.

Overcoming fear is easier than achieved. For most up-and-coming psychics, fear of psychic assault, evil, or detrimental forces and presences, feeling overwhelmed by the premonitions, or fear of a prediction of bad news are major concerns. Before you start facing fear, part of what you need to know is that your spirit guide/s and/or guardian angel holds an eye out for you; they watch over you.

Addressing fear of evil spirits and paranormal assault is very straightforward: if you're on a good path and don't set out to maliciously damage or hurt someone or live in anger, you won't be attracted to anger. Now, this doesn't mean you have to walk on eggshells constantly and let people walk all over you. You should and should stand up for yourself and defend yourself/them if someone has severely wronged you or another. Likewise, not living in negativity doesn't mean that you don't have bad days or negative thoughts to make yourself. It just means surrounding yourself with good people who are compassionate and loving, and not allowing these low moments of life to suck you down and make you worse.

There are many reasons why somebody would like to give you a psychic attack on your way. Maybe they're jealous of your success or friendship, or they're angry at you for something, or they're scared of you, or they're exploring and loving their dark side, and so on. Whatever the cause, one of the first steps towards recovery from it is to realize that you have been targeted for a psychic attack. Half of what the attacker wants you to feel is the frustration you feel surrounding your attack's signs, and that's what makes these attacks most successful. Knowing that you've been targeted takes that power away from them, and you can now take control. You're in charge now.

However, psychic assault is not the only thing that psychics have to think about. This is not to try to dissuade you from taking the psychic path or scare you off, but simply to make you more conscious of all the possible issues, worries, and dangers that may occur as you walk this path. It is safer to be conscious of what might happen and how to cope with these things than be happy in the dark until you have a bad encounter or experience, freak out, and become totally disillusioned with the psychic path.

A common one is a fear of being overwhelmed by your gift and being bombarded by endless psychic messages and premonitions. Beginners are particularly vulnerable to this because they don't know yet how to reel in their gifts. In doing so, strive to ask the world for help. Focus your mind clearly and state (in your mind) that you do not continuously want to obtain premonitions and psychic awareness. Practice turning your gift on and off, open and shut, energetically. When you want to start reading, concentrate your mind, and ask that the wisdom of the universe flow again. Before and after using your capabilities, close your eyes, clear your mind, and ground your power. When you are ready to accept psychic information, premonitions, and messages again, the trick is to remain calm and open and then to allow all the chatter and distraction in your brain to wash back in when you are ready to turn off your gift. The more experience and strength you acquire, the more you'll be in control of your abilities. It's all taking time.

There's something that many people overlook is that psychic readings will carry good as well as bad news. This is troubling to some psychics who find it pointless if there's no way to prevent this premonition from coming true, or who just don't know how to do it, and dislike asking the person they're reading about this unavoidable unpleasant, or dangerous thing that's likely to happen to them or a loved one, or manifesting themselves in some way in their lives. You may ask for this to be shut down if you wish to never receive messages, forecasts, or premonitions of bad things to come, particularly if they are fully unpreventable. If you are meditating and speaking with spirit guides, or concentrating your attention, and asking the world very simply, you may work to close these channels. Remember, however, that maybe these messages move through you for a reason before you do this. Tell, for example, you are very adept at predicting casualties that will happen in the near future. You get a feeling like somebody's going to die soon. Perhaps you have an idea of who, or perhaps you don't (which is even worse because then you can't really do anything or even warn the person or his loved ones).

You see this power as useless, but maybe the reason you've got it is that you're acting as a bridge between our world and the spiritual plane—world, and wherever the dead might go on their way. You can be a great comfort to the deceased, helping them to move over into the next life on their journey. This is purely hypothetical, but because your gift may manifest itself, it may have some sense or intent to do so or to show you/tell you certain things. Another thing is whether this is an obligation you want or not, and note that you are not obligated in any way to take on any kind of spiritual position or pathway.

Now you know a little bit about psychic work's risks, worries, barriers, and a few tips and tricks to help you conquer them and motivate yourself. Hopefully, none of this has dissuaded you from continuing on your journey to psychic ability and strength. Your capacity for a great power is there, and you will see your confidence increase as you practice, and your ability to combat others' fears, anxieties, and psychic attacks will expand. Eventually, people would not even think about sending your way destructive forces or energies. Keep up with your practice and adopt these security methods, and note that it is normal and just part of the psychic journey that you will have to conquer the occasional fear or destructive force slipping into your life. You just need to trust your ability and believe in yourself.

CHAPTER 24:

CLAIRVOYANT HEALING

You are definitely in tune with your caring side if you've chosen to awaken and improve your psychic abilities. If you are like most psychics who want to use your talent to support others and give them psychic readings, you can use clairvoyant healing, also known as psychic healing. People who desire to become psychics or a natural predisposition to psychic abilities are inherently caring and empathetic people, so it is no wonder that many of them decide to become healers and support others. This may or may not be something you want to do, but either way, this chapter will cover the foundations of psychic healing so that you can start helping others.

When you heal others using your psychic power, what you're doing is giving them and their energy to heal their body. You align and harmonize your body's powers and eliminate blockages to dissipate physical aches and pains. It is an energy-work method where you give unique healing energy to the person who needs it. Clairvoyance comes into play because clairvoyant premonitions also support psychics by giving them pictures of the issue to help them find the solution to how to cure them. Some clairvoyant healing images may also be sent by psychic healers to manifest their "patient" as safe, happy, and emotionally, physically, and spiritually pleasant.

It can be beneficial to meditate to begin healing others. You might also be visited by the spirit guide of that person, providing you with guidance about the issue and how to manage it. Focus on your subject, whether you have had a clairvoyant premonition, or you have been told by them or their spirit guide what they need specific healing for. It is better if the person you are healing is in the room with you, particularly when you start this healing journey first. Empty the mind of something other than what you're trying to treat. You take the unhealth out of the person's body with every inhalation, with every exhalation, you release it into the world to be turned into something good.

To help heal this individual, draw on Universal Energy as a strength source, as this can be a very energy-depleting process if you work without help. Visualize wellness imagery. Imagine that they reflect the picture of perfect health, from the head down to the toes. Start from the head, imagine them smiling and happy, naturally breathing, a light from them radiating. And if that part is already safe, work your way down the body slowly, picturing each body part in perfect working condition. The body needs to act as a whole—strong arms, heart beating steady, smooth skin, and solid legs that can take them as far as they need to go in life. Keep visualizing each portion to the feet. Imagine, like a dark spot on their body, the place that is bothering them.

Dissolve it with electricity, watch it dissolve, and disappear with pure light, leaving behind a radiant white glow. Then release and give this health picture to the person you are helping, through energy and clairvoyance. They may not be able to see them consciously, but the healthy energy and attention you put into them will integrate with their energy and their mind, revealing what they are working for to their subconscious. It will manifest itself as you sent it to the world too.

It is theorized that all physical illnesses can be traced back to mental agitation. Suppose an outside influence has a hand in things, of course, so that will not be the case. For instance, a broken leg is not due to depression; it is due to the tripping or falling off the subject and the breaking of the bone. 24-hour nausea is not due to an internal struggle with tension over a job decision immediately after dining at a two-star restaurant. It is more likely to be food poisoning, and nothing deeper is going on in these situations. However, it's still worth investigating a person's emotional condition with stuff like headaches, joint stiffness, muscle pain, digestive issues, regular nausea, etc. Is there a lot of repressed emotion building up? Are you depressed? Worried and worried?

Stress due to everyday issues or big decisions and events coming up in the life of a person? This can manifest themselves as chronic ailments in the body in physical ways that just won't go away. Typically some point of physical pain is indicative of blockage of energy. So, note that you don't just recover the body; you heal the mind, too. Consideration of the emotional state is always worth it.

There is no one alive who has not suffered anything and has no mental difficulties that create challenges in their lives. Although some more than others have been through tough times, every person has been through tough times, it does not invalidate the lasting effects it can have on the mind. Bear in mind when doing mental healing that everybody has been through different experiences and is coping with different things in their present life, so don't handle every healing session the same as you wouldn't heal a headache the same way as a sore stomach does. Ask the person to look into their mind that you are healing. What is their emotional condition, or was it recently? If they don't want to tell you, that's all right, just let them understand and be conscious of something that comes up and feel the force of it. As this happens, you could start picking up on a change in energy.

The role of the psychic healer is to cure physical ailments of emotional or mental origin. Focus your picture messages of the clairvoyant on what the individual is experiencing now. Did you feel depression or sadness? Send glad visualizations of them, surrounded by warm light, maybe running through a field of yellow flowers. Have you given up anxiety or worries? Imagine them at ease, with eyes closed, face and body relaxed, breathing peacefully. Perhaps they are in a mountain cabin with a cup of tea around them, nothing but nature. Stress and tension? Imagine going through their hectic day-to-day routine with light ease, not phasing them through the turmoil of their duties. They laugh and smile, and they almost glide or float as they move through their day, light as air. These clairvoyant images will help their subconscious release and let go of stresses that have weighed them down and will thus assist with any physical symptoms they encounter.

Ask the person you were treating how they felt afterward after you have completed a healing session. Have they ever felt relaxed? Was there peace of mind coming over them? Some sensations from the body? Did they come up with any emotions? And how about the levels of energy? Do they believe they've got more energy, less energy, or the same thing? Get input from this person and follow up a few days after the session to see if there have been or are still any changes. If you were treating a particular physical condition, ask how it felt right after the session and then follow up a few days later and see if the recovery had an impact on it, if there was any change, and whether it lasted. This may not instantly have a great impact, and if someone is changing but it doesn't last, note that it can take a few sessions—generally, it can't be done in just one.

When you are healing someone mentally, be mindful that it may take several sessions, particularly if it is anything more serious. As a novice; however, it's better to train if you're dealing with smaller, less serious ailments. You also have to remember that for your energy to have an effect, the person you are helping needs to want to be cured. They might even say they want to be cured, but they do not want to be deep down, or they are cynical. If that's the case, then they're going to be a healing challenge, and there could be no impact at all. Only make sure that the very first "patients" are not accused of not wanting to be cured because this could be attributable to the beginner status and novice powers rather than their disbelief or inability to be subconscious.

You can also cure anyone who is not near you in a clairvoyant way. They may potentially be very distant. This is characterized as a prayer by many. What you do is the same as if the person was with you in the room; to heal, you give them energy and clairvoyant images. After you've practiced and built up the capacity to heal someone physically close to you, try healing from a distance. Since they will not be physically with you and you can not sense their present energy, you will need to imagine them more intensely and more powerfully.

Picture every aspect of them, and as safe and healed, really put a lot of depth, aspect, and emphasis into the image of them. Visualization is the secret to distance healing, as you don't have to work with your energy. You can also loudly talk out what you want for them. The energy of your words will be released and solidified into the world, manifesting these health consequences for your friend or person you are trying to heal. Remember: if you rely entirely on your own energy reserves, you can easily become exhausted as psychic healing takes place. Tap on the energy of the universe; during your healing session, it will be an invaluable source of help.

If you want a test subject who is not going to claim results and is not going to complain or be cynical, try for your cat. They may not need healing, but try to feel their energy, and concentrate on your pet and especially your pet's wellbeing through meditation and see if any clairvoyant messages show up. If not, it's always a good way to practice having a sense of the motivation and emotional state of someone else, because animals experience things just as we do.

Hopefully, this chapter has woken you up and opened your eyes to the root of physical troubles for many people. It is of no concern whether you want to become a clairvoyant healer or not. This path is not preferred by all psychics, but they can dabble in it. And choosing this direction doesn't mean giving up any other psychic power element. It is only one capacity that can be built by a psychic. Practice, practice, and practice if this interests you—and don't forget to get permission from a friend, partner, or family member to practice your healing on them. It's probably safer to train with someone who has some form of physical disorder. Happy Cure!

One last note for this chapter: it is very important that you know that psychic healing is not a cure. Via clairvoyant psychic healing, you CANNOT diagnose. Let professionals diagnose patients! Psychic healing is extremely unlikely to fully cure physical illnesses or to replace medications for sickness and pain or treatment and therapy for those with a mental condition. It can relieve symptoms, get to the root of issues, get energy flowing and balanced again, and bring up the energy frequency of someone, but it should not be used instead of or as a substitute for modern medicine. Instead, alongside it, it should be included-they should work together.

CHAPTER 25:

PSYCHIC EMPATH AND TELEPATHY

Have you ever watched a movie where two people interact with their minds only or where someone reads the thoughts of another person to obtain data? Did you ever wish you could do this? Telepathy (from the Greek "tele" meaning "far away" and "patheia" meaning "to be influenced by") is contact between minds, but it's not quite how it's portrayed in the movies, like all forms of psychic ability. Telepathy can be exercised in real life, though; it's only subtler. For example, if you've ever been thinking about someone or just wanting to hear from someone, and soon after they call or text out of nowhere without prior preparation, you might have done so without meaning to. This is a way of interacting telepathically.

Without understanding it, the two of your minds connected, allowing the person who called you to make the decision to call—or maybe their decision to call is what brought them into your mind and got you to think about them. When something like this happens, there is no coincidence. In cases such as these, there are still psychic networks at work, just like psychic premonitions, everyone has the potential to use telepathy; it is only a field of our mind that needs to be practiced, but that most of us ignore or don't believe of because of how we were raised, the culture or religion in which we were raised, etc. This would make it easier for those who have been brought up empowered to develop the mind and seek psychic and telepathic abilities, but that does not mean that those who were not unable to succeed.

You may not be able to hold a complete conversation with your BFF using only your minds by using telepathy, but you may be able to communicate pictures, phrases, or emotions to one another. Let your friend know you want to try to interact telepathically with them to start with. This is particularly important before you start because you will both need to be in a calm, centered, and receptive state. Before planning to calm your body and mind, you should try meditating or deep breathing. They don't have to be in the same room; they don't have to be in the same space as you; they can be in their home, or they can be in another area.

Close your eyes and try to tune out all noises or background noise, and just concentrate your attention on your mate. Visualize them clearly in the eye of your mind-their nature, their appearance, their physical characteristics information. When this visualization of them has been solidified as if they are almost there with you, visualize the term, picture, or feeling you want to give them. Make it solid; make it vibrant in the eye of your eyes. Make it the only subject of your mind. Visualize your friend now, and visualize your friend explaining this picture to him. Imagine they will answer your letter.

At this point, they should have their minds open and responsive to your message, and they should imagine you in the eye of their eyes. Relax and let your message float toward the other person after you've done this. Let your mind wander from it. You should release your energy and concentration at this moment. Follow them up when the exercise is complete, and ask them what they felt or saw in the eye of their mind. Make sure they're not supposed to push any messages; they should just let their mind flow where it's going to and keep track of what might pop up.

Don't get frustrated if it just doesn't work. Practice and probably several tries will be needed. This is only one way to start training, but stay comfortable (both physically and mentally) regardless of how you practice or who you practice with, and keep your mind open and responsive to both sending and receiving messages.

In order to avoid the possibility of distraction or being snapped out of your concentration by unusual noises, people, smells, etc., it is important to be in an atmosphere that is totally relaxed, familiar, and calming for you. The best place to start is in your own home, maybe your bedroom or space you find, especially calming when you are just starting your telepathy journey, and you've just started to practice. Try your backyard or a peaceful park somewhere in a natural environment if your home is hectic and noisy, or you just can't feel comfortable there. Nature is able to help ground you and energize your forces. As long as this is a place where you can efficiently tune in, it should work.

The other widely known facet of telepathy is to read others' minds. It is harder to practice telepathy on strangers, so first practice with someone you are close to, a willing friend, family member, or partner, again. Be sure to ask permission before trying to read their mind. Mind reading won't show a play of what they think, but it will give you a vague concept, meaning, or maybe a word or picture relevant to what they think. Again, you want to be in an environment that relaxes you, the same as with telepathic contact.

Close your eyes, fine-tune everything, and concentrate your attention on the person you are trying to learn about. Get something easy like a banana to imagine the other person, and really concentrate on it. They can't tell you, obviously, what they're thinking. Until they confirm their picture has been solidified, imagine them, try to interact with their energies, and let your mind flow. For this exercise, they do not actually have to communicate with you or be on the same energy level because mind reading is more of a one-way street/one-man task, as opposed to if they were communicating their picture with you through telepathic communication.

Take note of all the stuff that flowed through your mind effortlessly—not forcedly—and check in with them to see if you got it right. Say you've seen the color yellow, or smelled banana bread, for instance, or felt disgusted (maybe they dislike bananas). If you didn't get it right the first few times you tried this, don't be discouraged.

An additional way to practice is to train yourself accordingly for someone you know, but then ask them a loud question. Tell them not to respond, but just think about it and process how they feel about it and what they'd respond to it. It can't be a question to which you know the answer or assume it. They would probably have an immediate response and/or thinking right after you ask it, so assuming you're calm and your mind is responsive, immediately after asking the question, see what enters your mind. To see if you correctly picked up on something, check-in with them.

After you've built up from these activities and feel that you're ready for a challenge, try reading your mind next time you're on public transit or somewhere in a crowd. Do this with as little discretion as you can. They want their privacy if you feel like someone's energy is really shutting you out and doesn't want to let others in. Let them be and find someone else who is more responsive, maybe. One common thing readers of mind pick up when reading minds is the feelings of the people.

Using telepathy is probably the easiest thing to access, and you've probably read the feelings of people telepathically before without even knowing it. It is necessary to differentiate between body language and facial expressions that offer you information about someone, and telepathy that provides that information. To stay impartial and make sure that telepathy is your only source of knowledge, try to concentrate on somebody's energy instead of looking at them/their look. You can concentrate on someone, try to pick up something from them, and feel a wave of worry washing over you. You can also pick up the explanation of why, but only in a vague way, they are interested, and it might take more practice to get this particular one.

Mind reading, in a way, is close to psychometry we touched on in Chapter 21. You try to pick stuff up from an individual: thoughts, feelings, pictures, etc. If you can get a reading from them without actually touching them, which would be particularly weird when performing in public in a crowd of strangers.

With telepathy, what is important to note is that patience is crucial. It won't work overnight; it can take a while until you get the hang of it effectively, so don't be harsh on yourself if you don't notice that you're good right away. You can also feel exhausted energizing after a session. Don't pull out your practice for too long as telepathy really works out your brain, and you might be tired. If a message doesn't go through, just schedule another day and try it again. Do not deplete your mental authority. And remember: do not look directly (if possible) at that person's face while practicing either telepathic communication or mind-reading, as facial features and expressions can cloud your judgment, mental concentration and force the reading or interpretation. Using just your mind, try to do it as best as possible because if you have it right, you can be sure it was telepathy, and there was no prejudice involved.

CHAPTER 26:

THE ART OF GUIDED MEDITATION

As described in the previous chapters, meditation is an invaluable tool to prepare yourself for using or flexing your psychic skills and helping you to practice and develop your gift. What it does is clear the mind and relax the body, putting you in a relaxed state, which makes it easier to concentrate on your spiritual abilities and the challenge you set out for yourself. Even if you don't intend to use your strength or practice, you can meditate—it can also be just a normal ritual or habit that clears the mind of worries and enhances the quality of life. Whatever the cause, in the next few paragraphs, let's take a look at some of the most powerful methods of meditation and its applications, and then we'll get into the subject of guided meditation.

Meditation is a way for the mind to relax and clear up from distraction, clutter, and chatter. It has been used for thousands of years, but it is now more relevant than ever. As our attention spans are shorter and we are bombarded at every turn and from every angle by information, movement, light, and color, it is vital that our brains receive a moment of total calm and relaxation, drowning out the noise and confusion in our lives.

You, of course, need to set yourself up so that you are relaxed and confident in order to begin meditation. That means wearing comfortable, unconstricted clothes and finding a quiet, peaceful, and relaxing space for you. If you would like to play meditation music, there are plenty of online choices, and if you feel like it would help, you can light incense. Decide how long you want to meditate on—

usually for beginners, a shorter 15-20 minute session is recommended—and settle in. Concentrate on breathing, in and out. Don't think or try to analyze your breathing; just let it be your priority, and nothing else. Recognize them if any thoughts flood through your mind, but then let them float away.

Do not hold on to any concerns or plans; just see the idea, understand it, and then let it go—at least when you are meditating. With no worldly distractions, the trick is to keep your mind open and calm. Your mind will eventually wander, particularly as a beginner, but this is not an issue—just be sure to let any thought go and bring your attention back to your breathing right around. If it helps, try to concentrate on one thing and do away with worldly distractions, you can have a chant or mantra playing in your mind. It will help you get into a trancelike state and get into the desired state of meditation by repeating a phrase, mantra, or mental picture of something peaceful. Pick something easy, something that makes you feel relaxed and unemotional if you decide to concentrate on a picture. This may also be a method for visualization.

For the duration of your meditation, make sure the posture you are in would also be comfortable. You don't want to get a cramp or have a limb fall asleep. This is a simple beginner's meditation guide to give you some context, in general. Now, we're going to get into a guided meditation, how to do it, and why it's useful.

One of the more recent branches of meditation is guided meditation in particular. It's self-explanatory, more or less. It's in the name—in your meditation there's some sort of a guide. It can be a person in the room with you qualified to direct you through your experience, or a recording of audio or video, or you can write text. The goal is to follow the directions and questions carefully during your meditation, whatever type you use, to reveal some insight to you and to elevate your energy. In the meantime, there's always calm and serene music played softly to help ease you into meditation.

The guide generally uses descriptive imagery for much of it, though some of it is up to you to determine. If somebody has ever heard you say, "I'm going to my happy place! And close their eyes when they've possibly built this pleasant place in their mind during a guided meditation in a stressful situation. An example of something from a guided meditation that you could hear is, "You're in a big meadow. Look around. What color of flowers are they? Is there a nearby forest?" These not only help to establish pleasant escapes and a sanctuary from the stressful moments of life, but at the end of the guided meditation, your choices are often examined to reveal more about who you are as a person, what decision you should make about something or insight into your current emotional state. Focusing on the body is another element, which could be used in a guided meditation.

The guide could tell you to concentrate on different parts of your body to check whether they're comfortable or not, how they feel, to relax if they're not already. They could ask what feelings you are experiencing in your body and in specific locations. This helps calm the physical self, which is also important as part of meditation. Driven meditation may be so calming that, during the experience, individuals can sometimes fall asleep. Try leaning against something comfortable rather than lying on your back if you want to stay awake for the whole meditation, or if you're watching a video or listening to an audio meditation, try to watch the photos the video uses or bring up an online nature slideshow to watch along with them. Just make sure that your meditative attention won't distract you from it.

During these meditations, the subconsciousness is at the forefront. That is why you can examine and interpret your choices while in this profoundly relaxed state to reveal valuable details. To this end, the guide produced them. The more you go into meditation, the more you go into this relaxed environment, and the better you feel. In this state, the mind is free and fragile-just as you need it to be for psychic work.

On the internet, there are several free guided meditations; you don't have to see a therapist or leave your home in comfort. Often they provide audio with a montage of eye-catching scenery and pictures of nature. You could watch the slideshow, or you could just lay back and listen. Before they go to sleep, many people want to listen to and obey guided meditations, saying it helps them fall asleep quickly and achieve a restful night's sleep.

You may also enter a guided meditation class or do one-on-one sessions where a live teacher who's in the room with you guides you through your meditation. You can prefer one of these approaches over the other, depending on your personality, but if you're uncertain, you may try both, live guide or online guidance, and see how you prefer or feel more relaxed. After all, the whole argument about your relaxation.

Not all meditations which are guided are created equal. There are many different types, and for many different reasons, they are useful. Some may be used to convey various things, such as abundance and performance. Some are used to reinforce and establish relationships, to better oneself, and to heal. When it comes to helping with psychic capacity and growth, the best ones to look up are those who focus on inner harmony and inner calm. Creating a quiet mind will significantly enhance your concentration.

It's uncommon in this era of technology to find someone with a longer span of attention who will hop at the chance to lay down and do nothing basically. Most of us will feel aghast or bored. This is not inherently a negative thing; there is no emphasis at the right or the wrong level. This, though, is a tool that's always worth dealing with. Initially, try brief meditations and work your way up. Do them before bed when you haven't done anything except to look at the wall before you fall asleep. In your set, this is a tool you're going to want to have, particularly as an up and coming psychic with blossoming abilities that need to be sharpened and concentrated.

You will find that you will significantly enhance your spiritual ability if you use guided meditations even very often, and your mental and physical well-being will benefit on top of that. If you don't always have the time, energy, or attention span to devote to sitting or lying down for a guided meditation, it's understandable in today's fast-paced environment. However, it would do nothing but good if you just make an effort and fit it in when you can, like before bed. It will become easier to integrate into your routine once you turn it into a habit, and it will come as easily as eating three meals a day and brushing your morning teeth pretty quickly. At your newfound inner stillness, you will feel thankful and relieved, and the usual noise and babble of your mind will become more diminished (not eliminated that's not feasible), reducing your overall level of stress as well.

CHAPTER 27:

COMMUNICATING WITH SPIRIT GUIDES

One element that we have touched on in meditation and spiritual work has been Spirit Guides and/or Guardian Angels. Another invaluable tool for the psychic is Spirit Guides; if you want to meditate to just ground yourself and replenish your resources, draw more power to yourself before you start reading, or whether you are seeking help/protection—these are all reasons to try and communicate with your spirit guides and ask them for guidance and power. When making requests or asking something of them, always treat them with respect. Don't ask them for stuff, but don't be afraid or embarrassed to ask for help, as we can't do it all alone. Treat them as a friend or mentor would do.

Spirit guides or guardian angels are not deities that you have to worship; they are a divine force that watches over you and guides you, regardless of the name you use the word. You don't need to be afraid of any godly wrath-they're on your side and wish you the best!

There are a few different kinds of spirit guides. Your guide may take the form of an ancestor or loved one who has gone over from the physical world, but is still watching over you. If they are an ancestor, they may be someone who died before you were born, but there are certain indications that a parent who knew them will tell you that their presence is nearby—for instance if you had a grandmother who loved flowers and flowers are a constant presence in your life, this may be a sign that this ancestor watches over you. Many generations of Ancestral Guides will go back. When you interact with them, you may not see your ancient ancestor's face, but you can feel their relationship and attachment to you. You could still be watched over by a caring loved one who died in your lifetime. This will most likely be someone who died in your life earlier since spirit guides prefer to watch over you for your whole life, but it may also be someone who passed away later.

Another common type of spirit guide is those who come in animal form. These are called 'guides for animals.' You will possibly be directed by several different animal guides in your life, each with something different to display or teach you—you won't just have one animal spirit that's assigned to you. Animal guides are also known as symbolic, or energies that reflect the essence of every animal that represents them. This Spirit Guide will provide protection and guidance on assertiveness if you see a vision of a fearsome panther while meditating. If you see a bull standing peacefully in a field, this could be there to help you stabilize.

Your spirit guide will not be an ancestor, nor be any symbolic reflection of yourself. It can simply be pure electricity, sometimes seen as bright light. A lot of people refer to this as an angel. It is possibly a soothing and familiar energetic presence that has been watching over you from conception onwards. Make sure that your spirit guide is really any force you communicate with. If there is some sense of darkness or discomfort, then the being is not your guide to the spirit. Your only experience should be optimistic with your guide.

Now that you know the basics of what a spirit guide is let's look at how our guides can reach out and contact/communicate. This may be the first time you communicate with your guide—you may not even understand what shape your guide would take yet!

Meditation is the go-to way for most people to touch their spiritual master. There are loads of guided meditations available online to contact your spirit guide. If you don't do a guided meditation, when you sit down to meditate, only contact your spirit guide for your only emphasis. You may also concentrate on the reason you want to connect with them if you contact them for a reason, but at the beginning, just concentrate your intent on meeting your spirit guide. Clear your mind, and push nothing. As in any aspect of spirituality, if it doesn't work right away, don't be disappointed. With the powerful goal of contacting your spirit guide, just keep sitting down to meditate. In a vision or as an image, they may not appear to you, but if you keep your mind clear and let it flow naturally, you will begin to feel their presence, and your channel of contact with them will become stronger over time.

Through meditation, you can touch your spirit guide, but often they can reveal themselves to you without you being in a meditative state or reaching out to them, such as a crow swooping down to stand directly in the middle of the path you walked down, eyes fixed on you, or the smell of your grandmother unexpectedly filling your nostrils for a moment or listening to a song you always associated with.

Often when your intuition strongly advises you to do something or not, it sounds almost obvious as if an inner voice is speaking to you (similar to clairaudience); it may be your guardian angel, offering guidance or warnings in your everyday waking life. You do not need to do anything to encounter this communication; just listen to the advice and consider it. Your mentor, in the world of the spirit, undoubtedly understands things you don't do, and you might not have the knowledge, so it's always a good idea to trust them—but at the end of the day, it's your decision. They are not rulers but guides.

In the form of a dream, your spirit guide(s) can visit you and show themselves to you. If you have ever had a very vivid dream in which a benevolent being (whether your deceased grandma, an animal, or an energetic presence) has talked to you, indicated you, or guided you to something/somewhere, and you clearly recall it, the next day, or at least you recall the meaning of what they were communicating and showing you, this was possibly a spirit guide visit. While you can recall the figures, you met, and what was conveyed to you when you wake up, you are likely to forget important details—if not all of your dream as the day goes by—so it's a good idea to keep a dream newspaper and write down in as much detail as you can remember when you wake up. If you have to run out the door to work, you can write on your phone in the notepad; there's nothing you need to be fancy about. If you want to keep a record of experiences with spirit guides, symbolic, and significant dreams, when you get a chance, you can copy it into a paper journal.

Reflect on a question you want to answer or the reason you want to contact them before you go to sleep if you want to intend on meeting a spirit guide during your dream. As you drift into sleep with this in mind as your priority, hopefully, that night in your dream, you will meet them. This is a lucid dreaming device, so note that it may take a few attempts to get this kind of power over your dreams.

No matter what form your spirit guide takes, and the reason for which they are there, it is possible through practice to establish a clear bond and channel of communication with them. Remember: if you feel negative in some way or are surrounded by any dark or harmful energy from a force that you believe is your spirit guide, that is NOT your spirit guide, and you should withdraw from them. Your experiences with the spirit guides should always be optimistic—whether they are very introspective, or if they are the spirit of a dead loved one, then maybe bittersweet. Your spirit guide and/or guardian angel desires only the best for you, and they can be a tremendous source of encouragement on which you do not hesitate to draw on.

CHAPTER 28:

THE BIGGEST PROS AND CONS OF BEING A PSYCHIC EMPATH

Chances are you've been curious about yourself or someone you love if you're reading this. Maybe you, or they, tend to absorb others' emotional content. Or, you've been able to communicate profoundly with people for as long as you can remember. Maybe you have a feeling of compassion that's hard to shake.

Or maybe you'd just been thinking about what empathy is.

And nothing more powerful than love. For another, a pain compounded by the imagination and extended by a hundred echos, not even one's own pain weighs so heavily as the pain one feels with another.

WHAT IS AN EMPATH?

Perhaps some kind of superpower that creates equal burden as it offers advantages such as the ability to read minds; being empathic enables you to perceive what others feel at a deep level as if you were feeling their feelings in their body. However, as Dr. Judith Orloff, an authority on empathy and author of The Empath's Survival Guide, states, the word is not to be confused with empathy: getting empathy means our heart in joy or pain goes out to someone else, but it goes even deeper for empaths. In our own bodies, we really experience the feelings, energy, and physical effects of others, without the normal protections that other people have.

No one really knows how it functions, what could cause it, or what an empath's full potential is, but the accounts of "empathic" actions are pretty convincing.

THE PROS AND CONS

It is difficult to say at first, as we spoke about a moment ago, whether becoming an empath is a blessing or a curse. Ok, it's a little bit of both. What are the pros and cons of being an empath? Let's talk to them about:

Pro: You Sense the Emotions of Others

The capacity to feel the feelings of other people is a pretty powerful capacity. You will pick up on that more acutely than the average person if someone is feeling nervous in a business meeting or on a date, and offer help. If someone is feeling fear, you'd be able to interpret it and hopefully help them either conquer their fear or get out of a dangerous situation—this might also help you to become more aware of a potentially dangerous situation. Furthermore, you have the potential to connect to others in an extremely powerful way. An empathy gives an entirely different sense to the saying "to know what it's like to walk in the shoes of another person." It is a force that has to be handled properly. However, if you can do so; as a result, there are amazing gifts to realize—both for yourself and those you love.

Con: You Sense the Feelings of Others

If you already know that you are an empath, you have probably seen this coming. Like any other aspect of life, the ability to sense others' emotions more acutely and experience them explicitly is both positive and negative. It is potentially dangerous and can be very exhausting, both emotionally and physically, to directly experience the feelings of others around you without the freedom to pick and choose what you feel, leaving you grappling with pain and uncertainty. If it's anxiety, depression, terror, tension, panic, or sorrow, you're feeling it right there with the first-hand sufferers—without any control over it. In such situations, becoming an empath can be very hard.

Con: The Potential Is High for Getting Overwhelmed

Empaths usually tend to be extremely sensitive. This means that not only do they have no filter to hold back others' emotions, but they are also irritated more quickly by heavy sounds and busy social environments. Combining these two factors together allows empathies normal in busy or noisy environments to be vulnerable to panic attacks and general feelings of overwhelm. Watching the news can also be really frustrating for the same reason—particularly now. Histories of heartfelt tragedy and devastation are profoundly felt, and sometimes too much to carry away.

Pro: It Magnifies the Potential for Love and Compassion

Your capacity to feel empathy and compassion for others, as an empath, is at a different level. One of the most daunting challenges in a relationship is always to come to mutual understanding. Of course, we will try to explain to the other person how we feel, but they don't really know how we feel. It takes quite a bit of time and a great effort to really put yourself in the shoes of someone else. The door has been opened as empathy, and you can not help but feel the full force of your partner's inner feelings. This helps you develop a degree of love and compassion, which is very hard for others to attain. This will help you strengthen your relationships and identify more with others, even with those you would otherwise disagree with. You know that other people feel and can find common ground, fostering great compassion immediately, which moves you to act more kindly and peacefully.

THE PLEASURES AND PITFALLS OF BECOMING AN EMPATH

Can you sense what people are around you? Do you feel sensitive about your surroundings? When you put your hands on someone, do you instinctively know where to go to support someone? If your responses are yes, then you may be an empath. Take the following quiz: How sensitive are you? To find out whether a natural born empath might possibly be you.

Blessing or Curse?

What it means is not readily described in terms of being hypersensitive. The pros and cons of becoming an empath are almost undoubtedly polarizing. Feeling empathy is a blade with double points. It can be both a blessing and a curse. You have the capacity, on the one hand, to intuit precisely what you need to do in order to make others happy. On the other hand, it's easy to lose track of what you need because you're so used to caring for the comfort of others before looking after your own. You have easy access to details about what's going on with the people around you, but it's hard to know your own mind sometimes. Some people would enjoy learning how to be more empathic, and others would enjoy learning how to maintain the best parts of the ability and handling the more challenging aspects.

An Empath Can Be a True Chameleon

I have this hypothesis that people become empathy as a means of keeping themselves secure in their universe. If you know what others around you feel, then you know how to change what you say and do to make them feel better to be around, both emotionally and physically, so they are safer people.

An Empath can be a real chameleon, a changing tone of voice, modes of conversation, body posture, and choice of strategies and behavior to make people around them feel more relaxed. The problem with this is that they sometimes lose sight for themselves of what is genuinely genuine and valid.

Self Treatment and Self Detriment?

Empaths prefer to take care of their environments as a means of care. This is a fun roundabout way to do self-care. It is unpleasant for an empath to do or say something that would make someone else angry or sad, so they frequently avoid conflict in order to avoid experiencing the negative feelings of other people. It's easy for them to lose track of the fact they feel insecure themselves.

I know that first hand because I'm an empath. It was both a blessing and took a lot of painful lessons from me. Without being an empath, I could never have been the healer I am today. I can tell almost instantly when I lay my hands on a person what feelings are contained in the body of that person, what problems they are dealing with, and sometimes, even what they think.

There have been occasions in my life on the other side of the coin that I was not true to myself because of other people's desires and feelings, sometimes much to my detriment.

So, What Are We Going to Do With This Dilemma?

I have learned many important activities in my journey to take advantage of the psychic gifts and to lessen the difficulties of being an empathy.

SEVEN IMPORTANT PRACTICES FOR EMPATHS

1. Build Your Shield Body

There is a layer of your aura around your physical body, which is dedicated to your interface with your world. Your connection to your planet is shown by its form and state. "In contrast to their shield body, people who are empaths also have" thin skin. We are more easily affected by our world when it has holes inside it. Visualize an energy shield all over the physical body. Seeing is just as full and radiant. Maybe you see it as a specific color. Some people prefer looking at it as white or as gold.

Decide what color, and see it that way, will fit well for you. Imagine the body of the shield as fluid and shifting... not static. Here we are creating a shield, not armor. It's nice to be versatile, because you can let in what suits you, and you can hold out what doesn't. Snap your fingers into a position to hold. Do routine exercise of this. Another thing I considered extremely helpful, to hold a boji stone around it. Kirlian photography has proved this incredible stone to seal the auric field if it is kept on the individual for three days or more.

2. The Center of Being

Imagine, once you have the shield body in place that in the center of your being, there is a flame, which is your pure essence. Focus your attention on the flame, so bear all your senses. Be mindful of your feelings, emotions, and thoughts too. Try this first while you are alone, and then do it with others after a while. See if you can transfer your consciousness from your surroundings to yourself and back again. Note that the two differ.

3. Don't Take On Responsibilities That Are Not Yours

A person can get so used to taking care that they can feel as though they are expected to do it. That you aren't. Without going beyond the boundaries of what you need to do to protect your health and sanity, it is good to be as compassionate as possible. You are liable up to, and not beyond that section. If you're an empath, maybe your perception of where the line is maybe a little flippant. Try sticking to it until you get to know where the line is. It will make your relationships all easier and cleaner.

4. Get Used To Being The Bad Guy

Empaths are also compassionate and loving for the outside. Usually, they get the advantage of people believing that sometimes they are almost sacred. It is easy to be attached to being the "sweet guy." It is not easy to cope with others' negative feelings, so it does not ultimately benefit them or you to think about others. It's not helping them shield themselves from their feelings. This prevents them from growing up, and it's not true; besides, better than a padded reality to live in reality. Yeah, if you do not do what they want you to do, people will get angry or sad at you or with you, but it is important to note that their feelings are not your feelings, and your well-being is not dependent on their well-being.

5. Develop Your Throat Chakra

Often an empath will know what they need to say or do to establish good rules, but it will be difficult to follow through and communicate it. The throat chakra is the core of personal truth-expression. Through the opening of the throat chakra, we open ourselves up to express our true needs and feelings, as well as to express the creative force that passes through us. Singing and chanting are some good exercises for opening the throat chakra, expressing your feelings and thoughts with friends, and meditating on the throat chakra. Some healing stones are chrysocolla, turquoise, lapis lazuli, amazonite, and blue lace agate, which help with the throat chakra. With them, you can meditate, place them in a medicine bag to hold or wear crystal jewelry (necklaces in particular).

6. Develop Your Root Chakra

The root chakra allows one to deal with being in the world completely. When the root chakra is open, we're completely grounded and present with all that's coming in our direction. If it's not available, with what's going on, we can be disassociative, afraid, and have trouble remaining present. The opening and healing of the root chakra allow us to release the fears within a shape that prevent us from our highest manifestation. Some of the exercises that help open the root chakra are: imagine sending roots from your foundation down to the earth.

- Imagine you can breathe in and out of your roots, imagine.

- The inhalation, the breathing of energy from the earth.

- On the exhale, release everything that does not serve you that is inside you.

Obsidian, boji stones, hematite, and red jasper are some healing stones that may be helpful.

7. Smudging and Clearing Regularly

If you are having problems with your empathic abilities or not, it's a good idea to periodically smudge yourself to remove the energy and power of other people from your own body. Showering, bathing, and spending time in isolation are other nice clearing strategies.

CHAPTER 29:

ALL YOU NEED TO KNOW ABOUT ENERGY VAMPIRES

WHAT IS AN ENERGY VAMPIRE?

What is a vampire for energy, and how do you know one? Relationships often reflect an exchange of resources. To remain feeling our best, we need to ask ourselves: Who is giving us energy? Who saps this? It is vital to be surrounded by people who are compassionate, heart-centered, and make us feel safe and secure. It is equally necessary to recognize the vampires of energy that leech our energy, whether they wish to or not. In some, positive energy can be rejuvenating. You're anxious about a work interview, for instance, but you relax the minute you meet your prospective boss. He's so relaxed and accommodating; you're so nice too. Or maybe you've got a good friend around you that you really feel loved for. These givers of energy are people to treasure. The more optimistic people you surround yourself, the more you'll draw them. There are individuals you must gravitate towards in your life. Getting a network of supportive individuals around you can also repel vampires of energy. It generates positive positives. Negative pull negative. So, your deliberate decisions in choosing relationships will make a big difference in the quality of your life and your energy level! In comparison, vampires of energy exude harmful energy that drains you. Energy vampires vary from the purposely malicious to those who are unaware of their effects. Some are overbearing and obnoxious; others are charming and pleasant. You're talking to a perfectly nice person at a party, for example, but all of a sudden, you're nauseous or poor. Or how about the co-worker who drones on how for the tenth time she broke up with her boyfriend? She looks better, finally, but you've spent. The bottom line is that these people suck you dry at a subtle level of energy.

Energy Vampires Recognition Exercise: Take an inventory of people in your life

- **Ask yourself**: does this person typically give me or drain my energy? How do I feel when I have this person around me? Do I find a rise in my level of happiness, or do I get in a bad mood or feel sick? Do I look forward to seeing this person, or do I fear it. Recognise the energy vampires directly in your life, and start assessing those you want to restrict contact with or remove? Strategizing how to be around energy vampires and the time you're able to spend with them is really interesting if that's absolutely necessary. In reality, schedule at least one full afternoon with individuals that give off positive energy and prevent energy vampires that drain you. Note how your physical and emotional health is beneficially influenced. Sensitive individuals, like empathy, grow around caring, optimistic individuals. It brightens their mood and helps their bodies to feel good.
- **Who are the vampires of energy?** Your life may have many variations. Energy vampire types include The Narcissist, someone who is self-absorbed and has a lack of empathy. The Victim, someone who tires you out to find answers for their wining and lack of willingness. The Passive Aggressive, someone who makes you angry with a smile and jabs that you don't see coming. The Rageaholic, someone in their general vicinity who spills frustration on you and spreads toxic energy. The Drama Queen or King is anyone with stressful drams that tire you down. Hint: never ask her or him how they're doing! I present energy vampires and tactics to fight them in Emotional

Independence and the Empath's Survival Guide. This is especially important if you are an empathic or highly sensitive person who appears to be very vulnerable to the draining abilities of an energy vampire. In summary, therefore, it is very important to learn how to recognize energy vampires in your life and then establish a clear strategy for coping with each one so that you are not taken by surprise! You will then own the moment and prevent the resources from being drained!

The energy vampires have control over you only if you let them. You can have empowered relationships on your own terms by taking charge of this situation—that means defining them and creating a strategy for each one of them. Many people become energy mampire victims because they are unprepared. So, when you can actively and deliberately approach this crucial problem in your life, you are one step ahead and have your resources ready to go when they're needed.

To learn more about how an energy vampire works and what you might do next, read on.

They Don't Take Responsibility

Energy vampires are often charismatic. Because of this charm, they can slink out of trouble when problems arise. They're crafty, and in almost any case, they can pin issues on someone else. In any discrepancy or problem, they never acknowledge guilt for their position. Often you're left with the guilt—and probably the blame.

Take, for example:

- "I can't believe that no one can get this right. What kind of humiliation! I just sat back."

- He started to get upset with me, and I really don't know what I did.

They Are Still Embroiled in a Drama of Some Kind

Energy vampires often find themselves in the midst of a disaster, flailing with their emotional and dramatic actions from target to target. They flew this drama onto you when they landed on you in hopes you'll absorb it, repair it, and get their ship right.

Take, for example:

- Why am I still the one everyone gets upset with?

- That is not what I deserve. I really can no longer bear this. There was nothing I did for Ellen, but she stopped talking to me. Why is it that not everyone can be as kind as you? They still allow you one-up.

An Energy Vampire Never Likes Being Overdone, and They Don't Want to Share the Spotlight

That is one of several of their narcissistic tendencies. They fail to make another person experience real happiness. Instead, they tend to harvest resources to meet their emotional demands.

Take, for example "That's genuinely good news."

"Today, I actually applied for a new job too, and with my resume, I really need some support. Seeing it done, do you mind?"

"You are just so proud! Just three more certifications to come and catch me!" They minimize your problems and play up your own.

Energy Vampires Feed off Your Emotional Energy

And when you're depressed or angry, your reserves of resources are diminishing. Energy vampires will transfer the focus of the conversation to themselves to drain the most energy from you, converting your consternation into their emotional buffet.

Take, for example:

• "I know that your career is not paying well, but at least that's enjoyable. You've got to help me find a new one for you.

• "You're super swamped at work, and I get it, but I really need to speak with Mark about this problem tonight."

They Love Behaving Like Martyrs

Energy vampires put their issues squarely on other people's shoulders. They bear no liability for their contributions to their problems.

What they're looking for is emotional help to improve their self-esteem.

Take, for example:

- He's still so irrational. I'm doing the best I can, but it's never enough.
- "This day was off poorly, and it was only getting worse."

For energy vampires, people who are sensitive and caring are prime targets. You offer an ear that listens, a kind heart, and limitless energy. Energy vampires use your own existence against you in this way, sucking your strength away.

Energy vampires demand a great deal from the individuals they target. This constant drain on your resources will affect your well-being significantly. Over time, excessive stress can lead to anxiety, heart disease, depression, and more. That's why identifying the habits is crucial, and then working on eliminating them. This can include putting up walls to defend against the efforts of an energy vampire or fully eliminating the entity from your life.

The ideas may not work for everyone. Try them, and form your approach as you go until you feel controlled and secure. Define boundaries.

Although this might be easier said than done at first, you can and should create areas of your life where you will not allow the entrance of an energy vampire. May not commit to social activities, such as dinner or coffee dates.

Stop weekend excursions and other extended activities where they will be present. At work, by not agreeing to lunch and not dropping by their desk to talk, you will restrict interactions between the two of you. Perhaps you need to start small, concentrate on a few areas, and then expand.

Settle the Goals

You can't change an energy vampire, but you can reshape your perceptions about it. This may mean turning down the emotional valve and not giving advice when they give you their issues. This may also mean that you can not use them as any sort of emotional relief either. They would want to reciprocate. Don't give an inch to them. Do not give them space if the energy vampire phones comes by or texts. You might tell that you have plans, or you're not feeling well. When they continue to interface with excuses and don't get the emotional energy they need, they'll look elsewhere.

Protect Your Emotional Ability

In order to know when they have someone on the hook, energy vampires use nonverbal cues. Your facial expression, the way you lean in, the way you clasp your hands—an energy vampire will take these as signs of investing. If you offer stone-faced answers instead and just give their questions a brief statement, you will not open up to their requests, and you can save your resources for yourself.

Cut Them Out Altogether

In most situations, you have the right to fully delete this person from your life. This may sound dramatic, but in the end, you need to note that you're defending yourself. Ultimately, you are protecting yourself, your health, and your general well-being by noticing these habits and attempting to put an end to them.

No One Deserves This Kind of Maltreatment or Use

Surely it is not your fault. Some individuals fail to take responsibility for their own emotional intelligence, and that's not your burden to bear.

SIGNS OF BAD ENERGY IN YOUR LIFE AND HOW TO CLEAR IT OUT

We prefer to use the word "bad energy." We're fast to blame it if something is not going our way. People that annoy us or seem pessimistic are always plagued with it and are loaded with it in ways that just don't feel right. Is bad energy really a thing, though? Does it really exist, and can it screw us up, really? Here's a look at negative energy and how to get the life out of it.

Is Bad Energy Really a Thing?

Although "bad energy" is often a New Age word (as is "good energy") reserved to clarify the unexplainable, nothing is solid at the very heart of it all; in fact, we are all made of energy. That is at least a half-true designation, practically speaking. According to Darragh Dunleavy, owner of Trinity Wellness, it strikes her like a ton of bricks when a room contains bad energy. Dunleavy says that it can alter the vibe of the room if people are in a bad mood. "When I step into a crowded yoga class to teach, I can tell if there is bad energy in the room the moment I enter," she says. "In my chest, my heart, and even my skin, I can feel it."

SIGNS OF NEGATIVE ENERGY IN YOUR LIFE

Often you just feel negative, and it is an indication that bad energy overcrowds you, your relationships, or your house. There are among these signs:

1. Complaining Unnecessarily

Negativity is always so common that you don't even understand it, and complaining is a prime instance of that. Complaining often creates more grievances, which is a loop of negativity. This is a sign that if you find yourself crying more often than usual or have trouble finding positivity in life, you'll need to flush out some negative energies.

2. Criticism

Basically, criticism is the statement you make against other persons. It's never a beneficial thing because while it can feel right at the moment, it almost always feels wrong afterward. You are more likely to get consumed by it when you create a vibe of negativity.

3. Negative interactions

Another indication that you are surrounded by toxic energies is when you surround yourself with similarly negative individuals. It's almost like you are drawn to them because the people who spread positivity appear to be living in some way in a fantasy universe.

4. Blaming other people

Instead of being the captain of your own ship, you choose to blame others for what's happening in your life. You have an inability to look inside yourself and look at what is really happening in an aerial way.

5. Everything feels cluttered

A substantial indication of negative energy is disorder. It's hard to stay focused when you're surrounded by it. Disorder prevents the movement of energy in feng shui from moving into a home, but in my own experience, disorder in the home often induces disorder and anxiety in the mind.

HOW TO GET RID OF NEGATIVE ENERGY

So, now that you realize that you have some negative energy in your life, it's time to make it clear. It is a fantastic first step to be conscious of low energy. To clear up the energy, there are a variety of steps you can take.

1. Declutter Your Space

This is one clear fact. If clutter brings bad energy, then it will make things easier by decluttering. Take action to eradicate things that do not add value to your life. This is a system that does not arise all at once. Pick a closet, corner, or space for an assault every weekend. Give away, sell, or discard papers that are not worth keeping. Make an effort to take the time to replace it with one that no longer adds value to your life any time you buy one new, either give the item away, recycle it, or send it off to the landfill if it's time.

2. Establish a sacred spot

Now that you've created all that space take the time to create an area that generates positive energy, no matter how small. With some of your favorite things, such as pictures, candles, incense, or everything that makes your room peaceful and sacred, consider an alter, zafu cushion, or comfortable pillow. Make it you're room of reflection, a place for journaling, reading, or any conscious practice that you hold true.

3. Surround yourself with positivity

It's important to surround yourself with positive energy in the form of people, books, movies, retreats, etc. when you're in a stressful space and it's time to cleanse. It's all right, whatever appeals to you, but just be aware that you are what you spend your time doing.

4. Instead of criticizing, inspire

Show them, instead of asking your peers how they should behave. Be positive and don't talk poorly about people or complain, rather than asking people to be happy and avoid gossip. Build positive energy by not only saying it but doing it.

HOW TO DETOX YOUR HOME OF BAD ENERGY

According to Dunleavy, the number one way to get rid of negative energy in the house is by burning white sage. When you feel like your house is overflowing with bad energy, it is a must to "smudge" your house. Research published in the Journal of Ethnopharmacology's November 2006 edition found that white sage would actually purify the air. White sage packages can often be purchased at book shops, natural food outlets, or farmers' markets at online retailers such as Energy Muse. Crystals can also be used in your home to help flush out harmful energy. Here are some tips for smudging bad energy into your home:

- Start with the doorway of your home after lighting your sage bundle and then transfer space to the bed, counter clockwise. Wipe out all the windows, the doors, the closets, and all around the room. You can also sage yourself if you feel like you're hanging on to any bad energy.

- If your home is new construction, you will also want to sage your home in order to eliminate any negative energy that could have been brought in by builders.

- Sea salt is detoxifying as well. It can be used in the home in a number of ways. Scatter it around the inner perimeter of the house, for instance, leaving it overnight and vacuuming the next day. To detoxify the body, you can also put a small bowl of sea salt in water underneath your bed overnight.

CHAPTER 30:

THE ROLE OF MEDIUMSHIP AND PSYCHIC EMPATH

We have spoken about psychic reading so far. We'll talk about medium reading in this chapter. What's the difference, then? Well, there may be no mediumistic abilities for someone who does psychic readings, which serve as a vessel and a bridge of communication between the spirit world and the world of the living, but all mediums have psychic abilities, as this is what they use to contact the dead spirits.

Mediumship or mediums may be a word you haven't heard before. As already mentioned, a medium is a person who bridges between the dead and the living. For them, they will communicate with those who have passed over and relay messages to the living. If you have ever used an Ouija board, this is one type of mediumship, when you touch or try to contact, the spirits of the deceased—while Ouija boards are typically used rather than anything serious as a means of amusement.

The ways of mediumship used by practicing mediums are when the spirit of the deceased communicates through the medium, and when the medium receives messages in a clear-sighted (or clairaudient) manner and transmits the message to the living. The medium is most frequently requested by a living person to try to communicate to create a line of communication with a deceased loved one because they miss them and/or because they want a sense of closure because there are unfinished business or unanswered questions between them. The deceased loved one's spirit undoubtedly feels the same, so these sessions can be very curative.

If you want to become a medium, an intermediary between the spirit world and the living, you will need to have a firm grip on the four intuitive forms (even if you prefer one more than the other) as the signals pass through, and you will interpret them through clear-sightedness, clairaudience, clarity, or explanation. After you've been practicing your psychic skills for a while and feel confident, this is something to try. You can always be on the road of a beginner; just make sure you've got the fundamentals down. If you believe like you are a natural psychic medium, someone who, from a young age, has felt the presence of spirits of the deceased, then you might already have an understanding of how these spiritual networks can be expressed and used. However, to become a medium, this is not a must.

If you know some medium, or if you learn that you can get in contact with a local practice medium, ask them about their art. How does interacting with spirits feel? When did they begin, or when did they first realize that they had this capacity? What are some examples of the intermediate interactions they have had? If there is none, you can contact where you live, you can also search online to read first-hand experiences from mediums. Just be careful that the person from whom you are learning is not a con artist, as the world of psychic practice is full of frauds that aim to manipulate people for money.

You must be in a state of complete relaxation in order to start the practice of communicating spirits. Find a place that is quiet, relaxed, without bright lights. Feel the universal energy flowing through you, and relax your mind, letting fade away from other thoughts that poke at you. Now it is time for the spirits to be called upon. Make sure you have mastered psychic defense against negative spirits and forces before you do this next step, as it is possible to inadvertently invite a negative spirit into your home (see Chapter 22 for more information). To further minimize the possibility of accessing your space by a negative spirit, think of a particular deceased loved one of yours that you would like to contact (this could also be a pet). That way, you don't extend your appeal to any spirit that happens to be around. They are not invited; only the spirit of your loved one is invited. Call them out loud now. Ask them in your room, and maybe ask them a question or ask them if they have something to communicate with. Invite them emotionally too. Invite in your mind a picture of them, very informative, and mentally welcome them into space.

Ask them a question you have planned beforehand if you sense their presence. You may feel them differently; whether you smell the cologne they used to wear, hear their laughter or a song they used to sing, see their favorite color or a piece of clothing they used to wear in your mind's eye, or a sudden emotional change where you feel warm and full of love. These are all examples to show you that in your mind's eye, the way you sense them might not be seeing their picture talking to you. Via images that need to be interpreted or through words you see or hear in your head, the way they answer the questions may be. If you answer a question immediately afterward, and get a strong emotion, this could also be a response. Or if they respond clearly, then you'll just know the answer. Remember not to force their participation or reactions, or make them up. Let them just flow, and if they're not showing up or answering any questions, then that's all right. Just continue to reach out and practice and stay relaxed. If nothing is picked up by you, don't force it. Release it and try another time again.

You can also try to practice as a friend's medium, and you can call upon their loved one's spirit, asking the spirit any questions that your friend may have about them. Do not ask your friend who the person they want to contact us if you really want to challenge yourself. Go blind. Ask them just to imagine the person they want to touch and think about him. Keep your mind calm and comfortable, and be open to all energies and messages that you can get. If photos or emotions start to pop up, tell your friend about them. You can go online to look up psychics videos in motion and see how this happens. For instance, if you're sitting there with an empty mind and all of a sudden, a man figure pops up in your mind, and then the color red, and then the Thanksgiving dinner idea, and the scent of cigarettes, you'd say, "I'm seeing a man, now the color red, and something to do with Thanksgiving. "I smell smoke as well."

Obviously, you're not going to know what this means, so ask your friend if it's important to them. After all, the message is not for you while working as a medium but for the other person, the one to whom the spirit of the dead is linked. If this is a real message, your friend will get it straight away, and they will tell you what it means for them if they feel like it. Perhaps the man was their uncle whose favorite color or shirt or car was red, and at his house, he often held a huge family Thanksgiving—it was an annual tradition of the family, and he smoked, which was a familiar and soothing reminder to those who knew him of his presence. This is an illustration of how an average reading will advance. You will hear words or phrases that you can relay to the living person from the deceased as well. Even if it does not make sense to you, tell them what you see and hear in your post, as it may make sense to them and be important to them. If not, then just carry on. You probably won't get it all right, particularly because you're just starting, so just keep telling them what you're sensing and making sure you're not pushing those messages. Make sure that they naturally and explicitly come to you from the spirit you have contacted.

CHAPTER 31:

DREAM INTERPRETATION FOR A PSYCHIC EMPATH

So far, we've talked about the deliberate attempts you can make to call for psychic prediction, but half the time, it's at the helm of your unconscious mind. Dreams may be a way for the cosmos to disclose significant messages to you, your spirit guides, or even your own subconscious. Anyone may have meaningful dreams, but the more you become in tune with your psychic ability and the world, the more these messages are sent, the more you can realize. The interpretation of dreams in all manner of ancient cultures has been studied for millennia, and it is still widely used today.

So how can you say if there is something your dream is trying to tell you or if it is relevant at all? Well, normally, when you're in your sleep, certain items or items stand out distinctly and vividly and make an impression on you and that you remember when you wake up. If you forget the dream, it's probably not significant. There will be a figure occasionally that will tell you something specific that you will know when you wake up. However, it is also not so obvious. Throughout the dream, there may be a sequence of events that occur or an overall feeling that may be correlated with some aspect of the dream, whether there are people or animals or something symbolic with which you see or communicate. Both of these can be experienced and ascribed to your waking life. Know that if something particularly sticks out for you in your dream, there is definitely something to learn from that.

If your dream involves a person telling you something, how they look to you may be as meaningful and significant as the message they provided. If you are led into a bright and sunny clearing in your dream by a deer from the darkness of the woods, the meaning here is easily interpreted to mean that you are very depressed and need peace of mind (or are about to join a metaphorical "storm's eye" in your life), but the deer has sense too. If you were guided by the person, you were in love with, or a bird or your childhood pet, all of these would put a different twist on the sense of the dream and how you perceive it. If you've been led by your partner, this might mean that if you keep going through this tough patch, you'll be rewarded—together, you're on a journey to that haven. A bird may mean anxiety or restlessness, a need for liberty. At this time in your life, a childhood pet leading you will make the clearing mean your past/your childhood that you have a deep nostalgia and longing for. As well as its innocent (non-predator) nature and instinctive awareness of the forest, the steadiness, and silence of the deer will tell you to keep your head up and keep calm, and you will get there. Of course, there are many ways to view these things, and in the dream as well as your life, it also depends on the other sense. There are; however, several parallels between interpreting dreams and interpreting premonitions, as you've already found.

When interpreting your dream, an important thing to remember is to try to do so without bias. This will establish the most reliable and most truthful understanding. It's also better not to use outside outlets unless you're really lost, such as dream dictionaries or dream a-z websites or books. You should explain your dream to someone you know if you feel like you're not getting the full picture. They can see the vision clearly, even if they have no psychic interest or have never interpreted a dream before. Tell, you dreamed of a bear fishing with her cubs by the water, for instance. The cubs are falling into the water and being washed downstream, but the mother is not trying to rescue them. The dream then moves back to the cubs, safe, and sound with the mother bear. You just can't figure it out, so ask your friend, and they're wondering if you've lately felt distanced or distant from your mom? Or (if you're a mother) if you thought like you didn't look after your children and that you felt inadequate? It clicks on you right away, and you wonder why you haven't seen it before. If you're lost BEFORE turning to a dream dictionary, always go to a friend or family member to help translate, since dream dictionaries do not know all the specifics of your dream, mostly have an ambiguous explanation of one-word symbols, and they do not know the meaning of your existence.

Journaling strategy has been discussed several times in this book but again, maintaining a journal of your dreams is a good idea. As soon as you wake up, writing down a dream helps you recall and lock in the information that would otherwise be lost soon after waking, and you can go back and read it even if you forget, and hopefully, it will invoke the memory of the dream again. As well as helping to recall, it will also allow you to keep track of and examine any patterns that appear in your dreams. If you think a dream is significant, write it down in as much detail as you can remember—it counts for something. If you can't completely bring anything into sentences, you can even add a little sketch.

By challenging it, another way to begin evaluating your dream is. Why did I see that person here? Why have buffalo been present all along with my dream? Even though my dream was calm, why was there a sense of uneasiness and discordance? What was the environment of my dream? What was it I was trying to do? In the dream, who was I? Why is it that the bright red bird that briefly appeared was so vivid? These are a few examples, but do not hesitate to ask any questions that you feel are important to your dream.

In dreams, one common theme that people fear is death. If it's their own or a loved one's demise, but don't worry, dreaming of demise doesn't foresee it. Dreams are rarely premonitions and represent your emotional state and metaphors more often about what is going on in your life and what you need to deal with. This can mean a major shift or emotional/spiritual rebirth on your horizon if you dream of death. You may be on the move, or on holiday, finishing school, experiencing a breakup, etc. It can also mean that a part of you died symbolically and that the works involve inner transformation.

Death also represents a sign of transition in our lives. In fact, in tarot, readers sometimes tell the customer they are reading not actually to take the death card. Look at who is dying in your dream or what, and ask yourself why. Why does that person perish, and what are they reflecting or symbolizing as part of my life? How does this death fit into my life's context? Even if the person who dies is someone you know, it can still reflect a part of you or your relationship with them. More simply, it may also mean a fear of losing the person. There are several ways to view dreams of death, and almost none of them suggest that someone is going to die literally, so put your mind at ease and do some introspection or plan for some major changes ahead.

Another common theme of dreams is being hunted, stalked, or assaulted. The dreamer will sometimes feel like they're trying to move, but can't or can only move in slow motion. It may be chasing or assaulting you by some villain, creature, or animal, or you may not know what is chasing you, but in your dream, you can feel yourself being pursued. Dreams like this are often closer to nightmares and can cause the sleeping person intense fear and anxiety, particularly if you know that your attacker wants to injure or kill you (or if the dream involves you being attacked, they are already doing so). In your day-to-day life, this can reflect anxiety or fear. It can be very literal, like being bitten by a dog and being terrified of dogs or being followed by someone in the past which has caused you harm. It can also be symbolic, though, such as being chased by your boss by whom you are threatened in real life, and you will soon be shot by terror. Or being pursued/attacked by an animal whose characteristics reflect things you're afraid of—for example, being pursued by an owl does not seem like a particularly scary situation, but owls are quiet, lonely, and adept hunters, so this may indicate communication or relationship problems or a fear of being alone.

Try to hold it up to your life's meaning, and really challenge and dig deeper into why that particular person sought and/or assaulted you with the intention of harming you. Specifically, targeting dreams will reveal weakness and a sense of lack of control in your life. Dreams of pursuit and assault may not represent outside forces at all and maybe telling you that you need to take some time for introspection —your thoughts may be what is actually "attacking" or "chasing" you, and the source of these troubling dreams may be inner turmoil.

Another classic theme to dream about is being nude or just in your underpants/improper clothing. A feeling of insecurity, feeling too vulnerable, and metaphorically naked is the clearest meaning that we can get from that. It may also be related to a sense of lack of control and anxiety, or it may signify a desire to be respected and a feeling that not everyone likes you, that others may judge you (whether this is real or not). Something else to remember is: this dream might reflect that you believe everybody knows whether you are hiding something or have any secrets. The bottom line is that these dreams are considered to reflect some kind of vulnerability, so take a look at what's going on in your dream or who's in the dream and see you naked or not seeing you. In your waking life, this is possibly a representation of who or what makes you uncomfortable. If it's not clear, just take a look at your life right away and think about places where you're nervous. Perhaps you are very simply nervous about your body and enjoy the comfort of covering it under clothing layers. There may be places you haven't even noticed. There are areas that you need to focus on and develop your confidence—a message that this kind of dream was trying to relay to you. On the other hand, if you feel naked or semi-naked good and optimistic, then this is a good sign!

At the present moment, you are probably feeling really secure and motivated in your life and feel secure as if nothing can deter you. Again, one of these dream's literal interpretations may be that you are very happy with your body and optimistic and not nervous about its appearance. It may mean you as a person are satisfied with yourself and do not feel the need to seek approval from others.

Falling is another dream that's normal. This is another dream that can signify a sense of lack of control and be overwhelmed in your life, particularly if you feel pessimistic and when there is a sense of fear and anxiety as you fall. In anything from work, education, relationships, it might be a fear of failure, or it might be just a fear of the inability to keep up with your life. It can also symbolize a feeling of disillusionment with something in your life, some part of your life, or anyone. Tell yourself exactly how you feel when you fell. Before/during/after your fall, was anyone else around? From where did you fall? And what else in the dream was happening? In relation to your life, try to answer these questions to interpret their meaning.

You've probably already learned that dropping teeth is one of the most common nightmares, if not the most common. At one time, almost everyone dreamt of their teeth falling out. Since this is such a common dream, several different meanings exist. One potential meaning of this is the arrival of a big shift in life. It is a symbol of their coming maturity and journey to adulthood for a kid or teen to dream of their teeth falling out. The loss of teeth is related to the loss of something/a part of your life. It would reflect the loss of childhood, with the example of the children. Dreams of falling out of your teeth may also indicate fear, inability to make choices or disappointment that you feel powerless to improve with any part of your life. If your teeth fall out pretty easily, you could be frustrated by something in your life or simply unable to find a solution to something. On the bright side, dropping teeth can mean success, and happiness is yours or will reach your life.

It may also signify a positive shift in life or a transition that you are prepared to meet head-on, or that is going to come about easily. It is by analyzing how you feel during the dream that the secret to deciphering whether or not a dream of your teeth falling out can be viewed positively or negatively. You probably won't feel inherently good about your teeth falling out, but if you feel neutral or relaxed, you might view this in a positive way—a positive step for the better or for progress on your horizon. If you feel terrified and worried about your teeth falling out, this could be something more troubling and trigger some introspection, as well as looking at what aspects of your everyday life may be triggering those feelings. Perhaps it is time to make a difficult decision or come to terms with an undesirable change in existence.

Flying is a famous dream that enthuses many people to dream about. Who didn't wish they could travel in their life at some point? The dream world is the only place where we can travel uninhibited with no equipment to support us. What does that mean, then? Well, the flying dreams are usually optimistic, for instance, followed by feelings of satisfaction and euphoria. This can be a way for your subconscious to ease some of the worries that weigh down your mind, as sleep is your only release from them (although we now know they can pursue you in disturbing ways into your dreams). An optimistic flying dream indicates that you are focused on achieving the goals you have in your life; whether or not you are close to achieving them, the truth is that you are self-confident and believe you will achieve them.

Emotional wellbeing, and peace of mind, may also suggest a dream of flying. It could be a result of getting out of something or completing a job that weighted you down metaphorically, and now you're free. It can also reflect authoritative decision making. It may also mean that from a particular angle, you might need to look at things or need to see the bigger picture. If you feel pessimistic about flying or getting nervous and want to land and be on safe ground again, this may mean that you are unwilling to allow any significant changes in your life, choosing to stick to your comfort zone's comforts, routine, and habits. In your life, something could feel out of sync, and you don't like it, wanting everything to return to normal. While it's hard to control your dreams, the next time you dream, you're scared of flying, try to ease up a little, and relax inside your dream. Enjoy the excitement and the rush rather than feeling anxious, exposed, and out of place. In your waking life, this can help manifest certain emotions in whatever area you may need to relax and embrace any change.

Being late is a fantasy that everyone has at least once. This one is usually very literal. In their life, career, school, a date, etc., the dreaming person anticipates some major event that they can not be late for or miss, and possibly have to wake up early and set the alarm. Dreaming of being late, sleeping in, not going off your alarm, or missing anything altogether is typical because you've been thinking about making sure you get on-time to this case. The dream will always be focused around the event itself, and you'll wake up happy that you didn't miss it.

A dream like this will symbolically tell you that there's so much on your plate and that you can't keep up with it all. It's asking you to take it easy with your life's obligations, and maybe take on less. In your life, dreaming of being late can represent a feeling of being overwhelmed, generally juggling too much at once and thereby creating a sense of chaos. Try to see what obligations and tasks you can cut back on and where you can add to your everyday life some extra "me time." From work, school, or your home life, you can feel a lot of pressure and demand. In today's fast-paced world, sometimes it's difficult to make time for yourself, but it's best to listen to your subconscious. If something can be shifted or cut out to build the space, then do it. The need for improvement is apparent. Just because you can multitask is not supposed to mean you can! Such dreams may also suggest an authority issue if you don't care or feel nervous about being late for a job or school appointment in the dream (or something with an authority figure in your life) or are late on purpose.

It is also a classic dream to dream of driving or being in an out of control vehicle. This dream has an explanation that is fairly clear. There is some part of your life that is out of control. Everything is snowballing faster and faster in your life, and you either have no control over what's going on or you believe you have no control over what's going on. Typically, the car and the road represent you and your progress through life. So something is taking control in your life path, and there's no way you can stop it. If you're not in the driver's seat and no one else is in the car, then it means it's your job to get things out of control and your job to get things back on track. When someone else is behind the wheel, be careful if that person is a part of your waking life as well.

The vision might warn you that this individual is a bad influence or is leading your path astray. It may be trying to warn you that you are being exploited by this person and that they don't have your best interests at heart. They could even mean to do harm to you. Do not let this person power your metaphoric car, and in your waking life, keep an eye on them. Note your experiences and the other person's behavior towards you. Dreams of out of control vehicles, however, are not always evil. If you are a child beginning to mature and reach the next stage of your life, then dreaming that you have to unexpectedly reach the driver's seat and try to take control of this out of control car (this is a common dream for kids because kids have never driven), this may be indicative of you entering the uncertain world of adulthood, unaware of certain expectations, and how to proceed.

This is particularly telling if the parents of the child were in the front seat at one moment, and then they abruptly vanish, and it is up to the child to steer the vehicle. This is reflected in their reality because many of the things they relied on their parents to do are now up to them to do. They've got more tasks. Tell yourself how you feel while dreaming of an out of control vehicle. Who is with you, or is not in the car? Are you solitary? What setting is it? And what was going on before / after the car lost control? In contrast to your own life, these are what to look at and keep up.

Perhaps a slightly less popular dream is a natural catastrophe, but the message is generally quite important. Dreaming of a natural catastrophe doesn't mean the catastrophe in your waking life will hit, so don't worry—don't take it too literally. Emotional repression is the most common definition of a natural disaster (earthquake, wind, lightning, hurricane, tornado, volcano, tsunami, etc ..). It may be a very general sign of emotional repression, or it may become more precise. A dream of a volcano or lightning bolt, for example, might reflect pent-up rage, while a flood or monsoon may unrecognize repressed sorrow or even depression. A violent, chaotic storm may once again symbolize rage, or restless hostility, and/or energy that has no outlet in your daily lives. Earthquakes will tell you the same thing, and they could mean anger as well. Another thing that might mean dreaming of a natural catastrophe is a major shift in life or some form of upheaval-typically a positive change in most cases.

Keep an eye on the four elements showing up in your dreams (water, earth, fire, and air). Think about how the aspect appears in your dream, what it's considered to mean, and how you feel about seeing it in your dream.

Water dreams are typically emotionally linked. A dream of water in your present reality is likely to tell you something about your emotional condition. How is the water flowing out to you? How do you deal with it, and what thoughts do you have about it? Emotional clarity, peace of mind, and security are signified by calm and crystal-clear waters. However, if the water is dark or dirty, this means that there is an aspect of your life that is undecipherable to you at the moment, most likely rooted in feeling, something you might have been wrestling with for a while and just can't find out. Dark and deep waters expose quite deep feelings. You may have recently fallen in love or lost a loved one or witnessed some sort of significant emotional event in your life.

There may be feeling that you are not aware of on a subconscious level as well. If you're afraid of water in your dream, you're probably having a hard time coming to terms with how you feel about something in your waking life and your emotions. Dreaming of a dreadful ocean storm or tsunami may mean that your metaphorical dam is about to explode. Repressed feelings are bubbling up. It can also mean that you feel really out of control for a portion of your life like you don't understand events that happen. Having a tsunami in a dream means you're meant to be bracing for things to come in your waking life. Dreams of drowning can also be a symptom of being unable to confront and deal with feelings. Water dreams can also demonstrate that our spirit and we have a need to cleanse ourselves. It wouldn't symbolize that your subconscious simply needs you to physically clean up yourself or take a shower, but it could imply that more of an emotional and spiritual cleansing/healing is in order, particularly if you've recently been dealing with some kind of emotional trauma or crisis. Or even in the past and those emotions all built up. Water may also be a significant symbol of regeneration and a new task or chapter of your life. You could come up with entirely new beginnings and new possibilities.

Rage, passion, affection, violence, flame, destruction, and energy are a few of the words associated with fire. Depending on the background, a dream about the fire can mean several things, like the type of fire, how you felt, what the fire was doing, and how you were involved. Fire dreams will also have, just as water does, something to do with rebirth. Just look at what nature does with flames. Yeah, it can be damaging, but to make room for new growth, it burns away the old. A fire dream may symbolize letting things go and letting yourself grow and mature and your spirit. A perfect metaphor for the good sign that the aspect of fire will represent to you in a dream is the symbol of the phoenix rising from the ashes. However, if anything in your dream is consumed by fire and you feel upset about it, this may mean that your waking life is consumed by your (probably more negative) emotions. Examine yourself for anger, addiction, envy, restlessness, etc., without power.

Try to find a safe outlet in your life for these feelings, so they don't build up and have a detrimental impact on your mental, spiritual, and emotional condition. The more the fire in your dream is controlled, the more secure your emotions and your life are. The more fire is out of reach, the more it can be a sign of major change or a suggestion to reel in some of your emotional outbursts and passions. If you are not someone who communicates your feelings passionately and outwardly, then an out of control fire can be interpreted as your subconscious coming with repressed emotions to the breaking point, and you need to let it out somehow, but be careful. It could have detrimental effects on your life to just let loose. Think about stuff and don't do or say something you're going to regret later. Maybe try some introspection and speak to someone who is trusted and detached from your situation or emotions, even a specialist, if you think this level of advice is needed. Fire is an impulse warning, so be careful not to be too impulsive if you are already an impulsive person, that goes double. Note, though, if you feel negative about the fire in your dream, considering its negative reputation, you don't have to fear it. Think of a phoenix emerging again from the ashes. In dreams, fire is more often than not a good sign.

It can be interpreted in many ways to dream about the earth aspect, so anything involving soil, the earth, trees, mountains, and nature, in general, as it takes many forms. It may also be less apparent to us when we sleep, despite its regular presence in our dreams, because it is still there in the shape of the ground on which we stand. However, this is not the only form it takes, as it is a very flexible feature. Let's take a look at some of its more symbolic dream appearances. Earth differs from the three other elements since it is the only solid. In general, grounding, equilibrium, and the material or physical domain are what it portrays. It is also a sign of rigidity, stubbornness, and unchanging nature. The one time Earth can signify a rebirth in dreams is when you dream or see something just beginning to grow or blossom out of Earth in your dream, or some kind of new development. Earth being the symbol of materialism, this might mean success and prosperity growth, which is typically financial.

The planet, however, is also the metaphor for the existence of Mother Earth/Mother, so this may symbolize the fertility or life richness. Being trapped in the mud or being sucked down and swallowed by the earth might symbolize financial hardship or a feeling of being overwhelmed at the moment with all you have to do in your life, particularly if that is accompanied by a feeling of fear. In some way, being inside the earth, entering a cave, underground space, or tunnel could mean that you are exploring and becoming more aware of your subconsciousness. You become aware of something that is concealed from your conscious mind or made aware of it. Typically this is a good sign and can be benefit to personal development, but these visions can also be terrifying. This can be due to the fact that there is something there that you don't want to face if you feel scared while going underground in a dream. There is something in your subconscious that you have hidden that you do not want to see or to deal with. That is what these dreams usually mean.

Less visible in dreams is air, like earth, than is fire and water. This is because earth and air are bound to be frequently in our dreams—like the air we breathe and the land on which we stand. However, as well as this less obvious appearance, it can take on other shapes. So let's look at how it happens in our dreams and what it can mean. Air represents knowledge, communication, and spirituality (although it can be said that, in one way or another, each aspect has spiritual relations, as they are all equally part of our world). The vulnerability can be symbolized by harsh and gusting winds that leave you feeling unsettled and uncomfortable or more negative feelings in a dream. Maybe you feel spiritually/ emotionally insecure in your life, or maybe you are not even conscious of these weaknesses. We have discussed flying dreams and what they symbolize, but here we will touch it briefly as it falls under the aspect of air.

More often than not, a dream of flying is positive, and if it is a positive flying dream, it reflects the peace of mind and a sense of independence. Maybe you have just paid off a loan or completed a mission or ended a relationship. Maybe it's a more philosophical explanation, but whatever it is, if you have a positive flying dream, something in your life has definitely given you great peace of mind. Count yourself fortunate as some of the greatest dreams people can have are the flying dreams. Air, like water and fire, is a versatile product that is highly changeable. A great storm or wind may signify a significant change in life, as well as vulnerability. If there's a lack of air or it feels hard to breathe, in your waking life, you can feel panicked, nervous, and exhausted. This could mean emotional distance/coldness, and/or loneliness or an undesirable distance from those you care for if the air is cold. In your dream, gusts of wind that appear negatively may also mean that you need to ground yourself and get in touch with reality.

Note, it's all symbolic—these visions of the elements aren't premonitions of drowning or being burned in a fire or being swallowed by the earth, or being sucked away by a tornado. If they come with negative feelings, then there is something in your life that is causing these significant and powerful dream messages—and interpreting them is a step in the right direction to figuring out how to get to the bottom of these feelings or issues, tackle them, grow, and move on.

CHAPTER 32:

PSYCHIC DEVELOPMENT EXERCISES FOR EMPATHS

Let us get down to business now. I will teach you how to turn your abilities on and off in this chapter and then describe four basic exercises that will help you improve your psychic gifts and refine them. The single most important thing you need at this stage, in addition to your ability to explore your psychic abilities, is a partner or a group of like-minded people.

GATHERING LIKE-MINDED PEOPLE

Having a group of people together who are serious about psychic development is one of the most important ingredients for your development. Ask friends and colleagues (with whom you trust and feel safe) if any of them are interested in improving their skills or helping you improve yours. You may have friends who are interested, but don't live near you, in improving their psychic skills. You can do exercise 1 over the internet, emails, or regular mail, for example, and you can do exercises 2 and 4 via regular mail. Granted, it will not be the same as practicing them in person, but there are ways you can practice for those of you without access to a large group of people. The key thing is for you to practice on people.

Until you have assembled a group of people who are interested in improving their psychic abilities, I want you to make a commitment to meet for continuity every week, at the same time and place, if possible. It's helpful if you don't really know each other well, then you're going to lecture each other. Previous knowledge about someone can interfere with whether or not the information you are getting is real or based on what you already know about it, especially when you start reading first.

Note, choosing people with whom you feel comfortable and who won't make fun of you is important. Our egos get in the way, which is enough when it comes to cultivating these gifts; don't make it harder for yourself by choosing mates you will have to prove yourself to. That sort of situation can produce an enormous block. None of us like to be made fun of or put on the spot, so make sure that the people you want to work with are not sabotaging your growth.

TURNING YOUR ABILITIES ON AND OFF

My guess is, if you're reading this book, you know you have some sort of psychic powers, but they're either hit or miss. Wherever you like, you can't call them, and they may come when you least expect or want them to. With untrained psychic powers, this is very normal, so don't get discouraged. Turning your skills on and turning them off at will is possible.

My students always tell me that once they have opened up their psychic outlets, they don't want to shut them down for fear of never coming back. They will, I can assure you. In fact, it is just as important to be able to turn off your skills in the beginning, so you don't develop a "third-eye headache."

You can only do a couple of exercises a week while you are just starting. It takes time to open your third eye and/or psychic ears, and it is like exercising every muscle in your body: if you force yourself too hard, you're going to hurt yourself. A third-eye pain, in this situation, feels like a tight band around the forehead, and aspirin won't take it away. The only way to feel better is to psychically shut down and walk away for a while from training. The area in the middle of your forehead will always be sensitive, but it will be particularly so at the beginning of your growth. Don't literally drive it because you're excited. You have plenty of time for your skills to improve. Pace yourself that way.

Now I want you to do a quick exercise. Close your eyes and concentrate on your forehead halfway through. Imagine that there is a closed eye, and next to it, there's a light switch that's currently in the down or off the role. Now imagine flipping the light switch "on," and slowly opening your third eye (yes, it's actually there). It may just open a tiny bit, or it may open up extensively. It is going to open up to some extent.

Visualize a zipper over your head now. Imagine unzipping it painfully.

Sit down now and concentrate for about thirty seconds on this image (of an opened third eye, and the energy over your head opened up). What is it that your head feels like? It could be a slight difference or a sensation that is very evident. Only have it known.

Zip the zipper back up and turn off the light switch with your third eye once you've done this. Close your third eye. Notice what it sounds like now.

Go through it now and do this whole exercise again. Turn your third eye on the light switch, unzip the zipper at the top of your head, experience the feeling of being psychically open for about thirty seconds, and then shut your third eye and the energy at the top of your head, noticing how different you now feel.

This is what you need to do to physically open up and shut down. You open your third eye so that photos, dreams, or images can be received, and you open your spiritual ears by unzipping the zipper on top of your head so that you can accept messages.

Knowing that you can monitor your gifts is vital for you—that you can turn them on and turn them off as you wish. It's also important for you to be able to understand how it feels when they are on or off. That will allow you to distinguish between being psychic and getting your own thoughts.

THE EXERCISES

Thirty-seven years ago, my instructor taught me the same psychic growth exercises that I'm going to teach you. Some of these are going to work better for you than others, but before you find the ones that work best, I want you to do all of them many times. Often one of these exercises could block you, but what I've noticed is that this type has more to do with the person you're working with than with the exercise itself. When doing one of these, if you think you're stuck, try it first with a different partner instead of chucking the whole exercise.

If you've assembled a group of people, you need to pair up, and then make sure you've got a new partner every week, so you don't read the same person each time. Count off to decide who your partner will be as soon as you're both present. If the group is an even number, this is the easiest. For example, if there are six individuals in your party, count down to three twice, and those individuals with matching numbers become partners for this week. Similarly, if you have eight people in a group, count twice to four, or ten, count twice to five. If you have an uncommon number of people (such as five), create a three-person "pairing" and have them read each other round-robin style so that no one reads or is read twice. You can do the exercises once you have your partner in one of two ways:

1. You can take turns with your buddy, and you can say it out loud as the data arrives and get input as you go.

2. At the same time, you should also do the exercise, both of you writing down all the details that you get on a piece of paper. Then you can check each other's paper and provide feedback on quality when you're both done.

In any case, be sure that if you analyze your partner's psychic details, you don't stretch the facts to make the details appear real. That will not help either of you improve your skills. If the knowledge suits, or it does not!

Before You Begin: Opening Up Fully

Here is a more in-depth version of the opening workout, which you can do before each session of practice:

- Lie down in a chair, close your eyes, and take a few breaths of relaxation. Ask the body to alleviate stress and anxiety while exhaling. Note any areas of your body that feel tight or painful. As you inhale, to bring calmness and relieve the pain, imagine your breath going into that part of the body.

- Let your body sink into your chair, so it feels fully supported.

- Visualize roots growing out of the bottom of your feet using your imagination, going down through the earth, and reaching at least six to ten feet into the ground. This will make the body feel grounded while you are psychically opened up.

- Now imagine your third eye, with the light switch next to it, situated in the center of your forehead. Visualize flipping the light switch to the spot on, then slowly opening your third eye. First, the zipper is visualized on top of your head. Unzip the zipper, which will open your psychic ears in exchange.

- Now you have opened up to Universal Reality. As you develop your skills, you will become increasingly aware of the sensation of this dimension, which is very light.

- Second, go to your solar plexus (the area around the button on your belly) and see a white light inside. Your intuition remains in this. Ask God (or, if you prefer, Universal Truth or Knowledge) to help you understand the truth of the data you receive and to help you interpret the data correctly.

All the structures are now gone, and you're able to do some mental work. Your third eye is open, your psychic ears have been opened, and you have your great helper, your inner voice (or intuition), ready to help you understand the knowledge that you are about to receive. Let's start.

Exercise 1: Names

You will practice tuning in to an individual's vibration in this exercise by concentrating on his or her first name. He doesn't have to have a full name. Have your partner send you someone he or she knows well by the first name. Write the name on a piece of paper, close your eyes, and ask the Universe to provide this person with simple, correct details for you. Remember to respect personal limits and ask for knowledge to help you realize that you are on the right path.

Concentrate on the name. Tell it to yourself over and over, either out loud or quietly. When an idea or an image comes into your mind, say or write it down to your partner (depending on how you do the exercise) and then go back to the name. Keep repeating it to yourself. If an image or thought of someone you know keeps coming into your mind, when you think of that person, write down the characteristics you think of.

Now tell your buddy, or write down the thoughts and pictures that seem meaningless or goofy. You'll be shocked by how much the seemingly insignificant information is very important. Your intelligence will actually block you if you start 'thinking' about what information you're receiving, so just keep concentrating on the name and writing down whatever ideas, images, or sensations come to you. Don't think about making mistakes. We just want to get things going in the beginning. The human propensity is to complicate matters, so remember to keep it easy and concentrate on the name. Remind yourself that you're cultivating one of your talents if your head gets in the way, and you start doubting what you're doing and thinking it's a waste of time.

At first, just spend about five minutes concentrating on the name. When the time is up, or the information stops coming in, use your intuition to run each piece of information for confirmation. It will let you know if the images, feelings, or emotions are precise.

Let's say, for example, that these are some of the things that came to you about the person: the outgoing, a sports car photo, mother, blue dress, pumpkins, Johnny Mathis. Take one thing at a time and rely on your instincts and ask if the knowledge is important. Every time, you get an inner understanding of either yes, no, or maybe.

After intuitively checking all the details, and feeling happy with your answers, give your list to your partner and get feedback from them.

Don't get frustrated if none of the information is right. The main aim at first is to actually open up your psychic centers and get the pictures and thoughts flowing to you. We're going to focus a lot on accuracy later, so be patient and stick with it for now. The trouble with the name you were given may have been, so ask your partner for another name, and try again.

When you feel pleased with your responses, hand them out for verification to your partner. Note that you are in the early stages of discovering how all of this works, so look at each scenario as a learning tool. Pay as much attention to the potential sources of inaccurate information as to be enthusiastic about the data you are getting correctly, and again, be frank about accuracy amongst yourself.

True psychic knowledge will not be fuzzy or sort of right, so if it really doesn't, don't stretch to make the data match. Do not spare your emotions from each other. That will not help you to grow.

And again, before you move on to another practice, ask the Universe to psychically clean you out. You will need to ask two or three times to make sure that you are cleansed of the energies of that person. Any time there's a lot of details, and I don't seem to be disconnecting from a single person, I think I've got an eraser in my hand and literally clean off my third eye. It does fit well.

When You Finish: Closing Up

When you're done with your practice exercises, you not only need to rid yourself of the people you've been hearing, you also need to psychologically shut down. After each session, do the following, which is a combination of the closing visualizations mentioned above under 'Controlling Your Skill' and the clearing meditation listed under the chapter, 'Protecting Yourself Psychically.'

Take a few deep calming breaths, close your physical eyes, and release any stress that may be sitting in the body. Visualize the light switch that is on right now with your third eye. Imagine shutting it off and closing your third eye. Then imagine zipping your head upwards.

Now, please ask the universe or Deity to make it clear to you:

> Please clear my body
>
> Clear my body
>
> Please clear my mind
>
> Clear my mind
>
> Please clear my soul

Clear my soul

Please clear me psychically

Clear me psychically

Doing this clearing exercise is really important because you don't want to take any of the people you have just read around with you. When you feel refreshed, take a couple of calming breaths and open your eyes. You are now back in this reality, and you can go about your daily business. Ask the Universe to clear you again if you still feel very spacey, and then ground yourself more by making one or more of the suggestions mentioned in chapter 23 under 'Grounding.'

Exercise 2: Photographs

You will read images without looking at them in this exercise. To start with, get three to four photographs of people you know well, and you can be one of them. Every photo should be of only one person, and ideally, without any pets in the picture, pets have their own personalities, which can cause confusion when trying to read the picture. Put each photo in an envelope and mark the outside with the individual's initials so that you know what image you gave your partner. Finally, share pictures with your partner one at a time, making sure that the photo is not clear through the envelope; if it is, send them the envelope with the photo facing up. You should tell your partner about the sex of the person for the first photo, but that's all I want you to share with them.

Decide whether you want to go one at a time, or whether they both read the pictures at the same time. If you want to go one at a time, decide who is going to work first, and tell your partner out loud what you're having or writing down on a tablet and handing it to them when you're done, as the data comes to that person. If you plan to work concurrently, simply write down all of your details and share those notes when both of you are done. If you are in a group of three, each of you in the group should pass a photograph to the individual on your right, and then all of you should read the photographs together. Start by doing the opening visualizations as in Exercise 1: open your third eye, your psychic ears, and your intuition.

Then keep the envelope containing the picture in your hand, and pray for simple, truthful knowledge about this person from the Cosmos, God, and your spirit guides. Spend some five minutes on that. No matter how foolish or trivial it sounds, write down anything that comes to you. If it seems like no more information is coming (but don't go any longer than five minutes), run the list for consistency through your intuition. If that sounds boring or time-consuming, don't get annoyed in the beginning. After a while, it will become second nature. You and your partner can swap lists when you have done testing with your instincts, and then give each other truthful feedback about your accuracy.

If you've completed the reading and received reviews, then both of you will look at the images. You might be shocked at how the person you are reading looks because it may be very different from what you saw with your third eye. Our minds are still working, and your mind might have put together a composite sketch based on random data you picked up. Don't be alarmed if the image you've had in your mind looks different from the real person. Focus more on your list of qualities and speak with your partner about them. Work between yourself. Share some data that will help your partner understand the photos, emotions, and feelings they have gotten.

Ask the Universe to rid you of the energy of the entity when you've finished discussing your readings. Then take the next picture, except that I want you to send the first name of the person in the photo to your partner this time. I want you to see the difference that it makes when you also have the name of the person.

You may find that with the first image, you are very accurate, but not so accurate with the second one, and that may be for a few reasons:

1. The guy you were reading isn't so easy to read.

2. Your pride got in the way, needing the second chance to make sure you were right, too.

Do not be too harsh on yourself if you don't get it right. This is all completely natural. You're going to go through different stages of being anxious, trying to be accurate, getting scared when you're right, and yet worried about being wrong. As we improve our skills, we go through a lot of adjustments, which is another reason why I want you to keep a journal. Write out the frustrations, enthusiasm, anxiety, fears, and aspirations of all your thoughts and feelings regarding your psychic abilities. Also, write those down if you're aware of any blocks, too. This is certainly a road, and "getting there" will take some time. Try to enjoy every move along the way.

Exercise 3: The Billets

Remember the character of Johnny Carson "The Magnificent Carnac?" The turbaned fortune-teller who'd keep a piece of paper with a secret question written on it up to his third eye and say the answer? Those pieces of paper on them with questions are called billets. There were billet readers back in the sixties and seventies who would hold sessions for the public to come and get psychic advice. Typically those were held in a large meeting room or church. There were a couple of them I attended, and they went like this: you will go in, pay your five dollars, and get a piece of paper to write down a question. You were to submit the billet to one of your deceased relatives or spirit guides, ask them a question about your life, and sign it in a loving manner.

When you were thinking about your question, you had to keep the billet for about thirty seconds, just in case, there were a few questions you were thinking of asking. Then you'd fold it twice to be sure your question couldn't be interpreted by the billet reader, and someone would come along with a basket (like the church collection plate) to gather them all and take them to the podium reader. An assistant would place cotton balls on the reader's eyes, then a blindfold. The reader will then reach into the basket for the next few hours and take a billet out, hold it up to his or her third eye, and continue to give the answer loudly.

The reader would often say something to help identify the audience whose problem it was by saying something like, "This question is for someone on the right side of the room whose first name begins with an F." You wrote this in spirit to your sister, and she tells you that the answer to your question is that you have to be patient until springtime and then you'll get the advice you're praying for. In his or her responses, the reader was always more precise, but you never knew what to expect. The individual would often say something like, "This billet was written by a person on the left side of the room, which today was going to wear a red sweater, but at the last minute changed their mind." And then she or he would continue to give the answer.

The reader never looked at a query once, but the skeptics all said billet readers had concealed microphones within the blindfolds and tiny mirrors, and that's how they knew who was in the crowd (oh brother!). It's your turn now. I want you to make your partner do billets. You both take a piece of paper and write to one of your guides or a deceased relative with a question. The issue you'd like advice about can be anything. Then thank you and sign the person for supporting you, just as though you had written a letter. For instance:

Dear Grandpa,

I am considering applying for a position at the sawmill. Do you think this is a smart move and is it a good time for you to tell me to do this? Thank you.

Love, Tasha

Fold the piece of paper twice and keep it in your hands as you concentrate on your question for about thirty seconds. Exchange billets after you've both done this.

Before attempting to read the billets mentally, make sure that both of you do the opening exercises mentioned above under "Before You Begin: Open Up Entirely." Then, without looking at the billets, close your eyes and either hold the billet up to your third eye, like Johnny Carson or hold the billet in your hands and just concentrate your attention. Ask God or your guides to help you with simple, specific details that will help answer the question of this individual. As pictures, ideas, and feelings begin to arrive, write them down, either on the billet's outside or on a separate piece of paper. Ask if there are more data for this query any time the data stops coming.

Students often groan over billets, but this is the talk of their ego. They feel like they have no influence over the reading result because they don't know what the issue is. Actually, not understanding the question is what makes this such a successful exercise, as it trains you on how to be an open knowledge source.

Anything that comes to you write down. Don't believe that something is dumb or trivial. Know, paying attention to everything is the best way to understand. At first, it is trial and error. If you are doing it right or doing it wrong, always learn from it!

Recall partnering with your partner too. Don't play the psychic stump by attempting to confuse your partner with false or unimportant questions. Together you are in this. Ask authentic billet questions and offer truthful feedback on the responses. Make sure to clear yourself before doing another one when you're done with one billet.

If your partner's answer to your question just doesn't seem to suit, there may be two things going on.

1. If you were thinking of writing two questions, the answer you got could relate to the other question you were going to ask.
2. It might only mean that your partner wasn't getting the correct details.

I suggest only doing a few per session at the beginning of these exercises. You should work on doing something, but remember, it's a phase, and you don't want a headache of the third eye. When you have chosen to do billets for the day, do the closing exercise mentioned above under "When You Finish: Close Up."

Exercise 4: Psychometry

Most psychologists do the psychometry. This is holding a personal item, such as jewelry, clothes, or a favorite toy, and reading it. Everything we have and use—our clothes and furniture, our offices and homes, our vehicles and toys and our jewelry in particular—have our vibes in them. When psychics read an object, metal is chosen as it retains the energy of people or vibrates longer than anything else. Psychometry is used by many psychics who work for police attempting to find a missing person.

I want you to bring a few pieces of jewelry for your partner to read for this next exercise. One-piece may be yours, but a friend or relative you know well needs to belong to the others. If possible, stop antique jewelry. It can be difficult to read secondhand jewelry because it has more than one person's vibes in it, which will make it difficult to check the details you get.

By the way, if you're someone who loves antique jewelry, I'd recommend that you sage it after you buy it. For a few minutes, burn some sage and keep the item in the smoke, asking the Universe to rid it of all the vibes it contains. For psychic individuals, this is extremely important because we are ultrasensitive to start with, and wearing someone else's vibes all day can literally drain our energy. I often recommend that you sage a new piece of jewelry simply because it might have been treated by several people before you purchased it.

Open up psychically using the visualization mentioned above under "Before You Begin: Opening Up Entirely" before beginning the exercise.

Exchange one single piece of jewelry with your partner after you've done it. Close your eyes, and keep the jewelry in your hands. Ask the jewelry piece to tell you what details it contains about the person wearing it. Write it down on a piece of paper as the data begins to arrive. No matter how dumb or insignificant it can seem, remember not to censor the data. Let it all flow into you. If your pride gets in the way, and you start to think about being wrong, remember that making mistakes is all right and that this is how you learn to distinguish between important and insignificant data.

When you feel you've done obtaining information, run it all for confirmation through your intuition, and then share the information with your partner. Be sure to get truthful input from each other, before moving on to another piece of jewelry, note to clear yourself. "When the psychometry exercises are done, be sure to psychically shut down using the above closing exercises under." When You Finish: Close Up.

CHAPTER 33:

HOW TO CONTINUE WITH YOUR PSYCHIC EMPATH DEVELOPMENT

I got an email once from a woman who said she was coming up for a week's holiday and wanted to know if I was going to teach her and her niece how to improve their psychic skills. Needless to say, her request made me feel a little flabbergasted. Psychical growth takes years of practice, not weeks of practice.

If you ever saw John Edward or James Van Praagh on TV, you might have noted that they all humbly say they can do what they do. What is rarely discussed is how long each of them took to cultivate their talents and how and what they did to achieve the stage they are at today. Indeed, as they will tell you in their books, it took them both many years of practice to understand and fine-tune their gifts.

If your ambition is to become a professional psychologist, note that there are many important things you need to learn and master—both personal and psychological—to achieve that goal: understanding, how to communicate with people, learning how to listen to your instructions, improving consistency, taking good physical care of yourself, remaining grounded in this reality and preserving the norm.

It is a natural phase to improve your skills. It's a path you'll learn a lot of wisdom along. Don't try to get along with it or take shortcuts. Accept what you are going through right now as just what you should be going through, and it will come when you are ready for the next stage of growth. Only believe me.

READING AND MEDITATION

I want you to spend a minimum of five minutes sitting in silence, meditating and concentrating on the white light deep within the region of your solar plexus on the days when you do not perform the exercises. This is a healthy discipline for everybody to study. Feel the calmness and comfort of this light and the wisdom inside it when you're focused on the light. Keep coming back to the sun if your mind wanders.

You should ask your guides to make themselves known to you while sitting in silence. Ask if they have some guide or advice about your life for you. Tell God to show yourself to you. When your mind begins wandering, concentrate on the white light.

Extend the time when you feel more comfortable meditating. The longer you spend with your inner voice (God) and your guides in silent contact, the stronger the connection will become. You may want to spend more time meditating on the light as you continue to develop spiritually, and I encourage you to do so. This is one of the strongest ways for us to create contact with God in consciousness.

Is the Silence Too Quiet for You?

If you find that you have a hard time sitting in silence and focusing, that doesn't mean that meditation isn't for you. Go ahead and build whatever environment makes you feel relaxed if you like getting some background noise. Don't think about it yourself. My brother Michael usually has some sort of background noise when he meditates or does psychic readings, like a radio or TV playing low since he claims noises help him hear spirits more easily. I once had a student who was still sitting by the air-conditioner in the classroom, humming because the quiet was too noisy for her while she was doing the exercises. Experiment to see how best works for you.

You can also keep reading about psychics and psychic development, in addition to doing the exercises in this book and meditating every day. I just want to warn you that you get too many details too quickly. This may keep you trapped in your head and can cause you to expect perfectionism; both are counterproductive. In reality, it's as important when you read something as what you read. Select writers you've heard of and trust, then decide if the timing is right for you to read them. When picking out the correct books for your needs, a significant rule of thumb is to run them through your intuition. Your intuition knows what your needs are and where you are in your psychological growth and will direct you to the books that you are ready for next. It is never going to steer you wrong. For a shortlist of recommended books and audiocassettes, see the end of this book.

Your Level Of Development Will Change Continually

Patience, practice, and respecting the process are the three most significant keys to your success. I also want to inspire you, on the other hand, not to be content with the degree you've risen to. I've never remained at the same pace for more than two years in my years as a psychic. My psychic gifts have continued to grow to a much deeper level as I constantly open myself up to what is possible. If you stick with it, so will your gifts.

I was doing five-minute readings for friends at the beginning. I was able to do fifteen-minute readings over time. They then stretched to thirty minutes, and my readings now run forty-five minutes to an hour.

The readings changed again when I got on my spiritual journey and began establishing my relationship with God. Deeper data began to come in. I was able to channel knowledge that assisted people in their own emotional recovery as I worked on my own emotional problems through counseling and twelve-step programs. When I got my own health in order, I began to more clearly read the health of other people. When I began working through hypnosis with my own soul, my mind opened up to the possibilities of working with people's souls, and the readings became more relevant to the purpose of their lives.

One of my students once called this phase having an "upgrade," and I get such a kick out of this concept because it's such a great way to explain the phases we're going through in our growth when we're about to advance to a new stage. From time to time, you will find that you are psychically shut down entirely. As I was typing this, the picture that just came to me was of a water tower with a massive tarp thrown over it that I drove by the other day. It was undergoing repairs, and you'll feel like someone has put a tarp on your skills as you go through these times, and you're under renovation, so to speak. When this happens, the third eye and psychic ears experience an internal change, and no matter how much you try to use or exercise the talents, you won't be able to. When you get the new changes to your program during these downtimes, you're going to have to mentally hang a "closed for business" sign on yourself. Just keep busy with your life while you're in one of those moments. Go to your movies. The yard work. Hang around with your buddies. Go walking. Do stuff that makes your body feel grounded. Get your closets swept. Do all of that stuff that you put off when improving your psychic skills.

I wish I could objectively tell you what happens to our "psychic pieces" when we're shut down, but I can't. I can guarantee you that when your gifts open again, they'll be better, and you'll feel "upgraded" for sure.

You'll also note that when you're going through an emotionally tough time, your abilities could shut off, or there's some sort of challenge you're facing. As a way of shielding us from so much coming at us on a psychic level, our abilities shut down. Be patient, and just know that when you are ready for them, your gifts will open up.

There Are Infinite Possibilities

Opening up your third eye and psychic ears and getting tuned during the day to your instincts will generate infinite possibilities in your life. Throughout the day, you can connect with God. From your spirit guides, you will get helpful advice. When standing in your kitchen, you'll see heaven and be able to connect with your loved ones who died.

If you want to and be mindful of other solar systems, you will be able to see aliens. Via mental telepathy, you can connect with others as often, if not more, than you do verbally. If you like, you'll be able to do remote viewing. Could you see auras? You would be able to see illness in humans before they even know it. When you understand how to be emotionally distant, you'll be able to see your own future.

There are so many ways your talents can manifest themselves. Here are four fields I would like to discuss in more depth: reading past lives, connecting with the dead, ghostbusting, and finding people who are missing.

Reading Past Lives

The first time I got an image of a past life, I'll never forget. I had to be staring at those pictures for a good two to three minutes as my mind was trying to acknowledge what I saw. I didn't believe in reincarnation at that point in my psychic development, so my intellect was trying to come up with some possible interpretation of the images other than that they reflected a past life.

A friend had asked me to mingle with her partner in her relationship to see if I could get some details that would help her understand why they had so many problems. In order to settle their disagreements, she also wanted to know what she should do.

The first photo came from the old doctor's office, and I saw a woman wearing a nurse's uniform. Even though this nurse didn't look like a friend of mine, I knew this was her on a psychic level. The next photo was a drunken doctor, passing out at his desk, followed all the way by a photo of her surrounding him with patients. I could see she had a friendship with him that was love/hate. My guides said she loved him, but despised his drinking, and every day she would search his office and home for bottles of whiskey and then pour them out.

The aspect that bothered me so much was that all these pictures appeared as if they were set in the 1800s. Since I did not want to entertain reincarnation thoughts, my mind became more and more obsessed with trying to find some more "rational" explanation. My guides at one point told me to just relax and open up to the details. They said later I could manage my own feelings of disbelief, but that I needed to give this knowledge to my friend for now because it would help her know how to fix their big conflicts. I agreed to take their advice and set aside my "things" so that more information could continue to be passed on by the guides.

They said that in her former life, my friend had been very judgmental about the alcoholism of her boyfriend, which is why she was an alcoholic in this lifetime. The other major problem was that she still took care of him, and he didn't want to be looked after. In this lifetime, he, too, was suffering from alcoholism, and he wanted to be alone, but she mothered him to the point of smothering him, never believing he could do it on his own. By feeling wanted, she gained her self-worth, and she didn't want to give it up. She had a lot of anger toward him that she didn't understand and still felt like he never understood "everything I've done for you." She resented him, even more, every time he gained more freedom from her.

After that, the guides gave some great advice to my friend as to how she and her boyfriend could solve their disputes, and the experience really opened my eyes to the reincarnation reality that I soon came to believe in. I've seen many past lives since then, and it's likely you'll get past-life data at some point, whether or not you embrace reincarnation, and you need to learn how to recognize it.

The photos may not look new, and they may seem very old as well as if you are being pulled back in time by your guides. You can also get an old musty scent, which will mean that what you see happened a long time ago. In time, you will automatically come to remember memories from past-life. Your guides will automatically send you the dates sometimes, and sometimes you will have to ask for them. You should ask the whereabouts of past life and ask your guides to recognize the people in the photos. Usually, the pictures just represent the primary individuals you are interacting within this lifetime. Often your guides may feel that not knowing who he or she was in a previous lifetime is best for the person, and they will not share that knowledge. Go ahead and ask all the questions you want but note that your guides have the final say as to what details the experience individual can handle.

Speak to the Dead

As you grow your abilities, you will find that your ability manifests through mediumship, or communicates with the deceased loved ones of people. This happened to Nikki, my niece. She was channeling healing to people, and slowly, one by one, the deceased relatives of people began appearing in her healing room. She didn't know what to do at first because the person hadn't shown any desire to hear from her deceased relatives, but she still wanted to relay their messages. She soon noticed that the messages were really important to others and that it was part of their healing to get these messages in, so she now uses her gifts in this way as well.

Do not be naïve about it if this happens to you. The reality is not informed by any spirit who appears to be someone's deceased loved one. I've seen earthbound spirits try this way to mess with humans, so you need to be insightful and firm. Only tell the spirit that you want some form of evidence that will affirm the identity of the spirit. Then, if the spirit sends you a letter, don't censor it or edit it, just pass it on as accurately as possible so that the client can judge its validity. If someone came across a medium pretending to be my father and sent me a really eloquent message—like "Hi, I'm the father of Echo. Please tell my caring daughter that all her work makes me very happy. I'd be skeptical because my dad doesn't speak that way. The message from my father will sound more like, "Hey babe, this is your ol guy. Keep up with a good job."

If you are channeling a deceased loved one, be very specific in relaying the message language and then check that the individual sounds right with your friend or client. Ask the spirit to give you some specific proof of who they are, if your client is still not sure. Don't embrace generalities; tell them the details you want. And if you come to believe that the message is not real, get rid of the earth-bound spirit by asking them to move on into the light. Recall also that when we go over to the other side, our appearance changes. Our souls usually tend to look younger as soon as we die. For example, if someone's father had gray hair when he passed away, but when he was younger, he had black hair, his soul might now psychically appear to you to have black hair. If he was very overweight when he died, then he probably won't look like that now because he doesn't exist in that overweight body any longer. He is pure energy now. Suppose you would like more details about the soul after leaving the physical body. This will give you a lot of useful knowledge about the future of life, death, life after death, and heaven for the soul.

Ghostbusters

One of the "perks" of growing your third eye is that you'll start seeing spirits and other dimensions at some point. You will usually only see little white lights, similar to fireflies, from the corners of your eyes at first. You will start seeing "blobs of energy" over time, and this could take years. These will eventually become more pronounced types of energy equivalent to a human form. Initially, you can see half of them, or you may see entirely materialized spirits. Ultimately you'll learn to differentiate between deities, angels, guides, and deities or ghosts on earth. It's been my experience that if your talent is to clear these earth-bound spirits or ghosts from homes and businesses, you'll be able to tap into them very quickly.

It takes a lot more than a couple of pages of information to show you how to clear homes of unwanted spirits, so if that is something you feel called to do, I would certainly recommend you get a copy of my books Relax, It's just a Ghost and Dear Echo. In both books, the whole subject of ghosts is discussed extensively.

Finding Missing People

My students also tell me that they are most interested in improving their skills in order to help the police locate children who are missing. If you're planning to do this with your gifts, then there is some stuff you need to remember.

The irony of wanting to find missing people (especially children) is that we're doing it because we care, and yet in order to be an effective instrument for information, we have to completely detach our emotions to the point where we don't care what we see. In other words, with our psychic eyes and ears open and our hearts on hold, we must go in. If you go in with your heart wide open, you have lost your objectivity, wanting to find someone really badly, and your care will block any "negative" information from coming in.

What you've got to do is remove your thoughts and remain that way. Get the name of the individual and deal with that as long as possible until you bring in other items like photos or material belongings to read. Something as simple as a toy or an adorable picture of the child will open up your emotions, and your objectivity will go out the window.

If the missing person's relatives or friends have called on your assistance, tell them to keep the details to a minimum. Ask them not to "lavish" you with the whole story until after you've given them all the information you can get. People want to share all that they can, but you need to walk a fine line: the more you know about the missing person's circumstances, or of the fears of the missing person's family, the harder it will be for you to maintain the emotional distance you need to receive the information.

Working with the Police

So often, when there's a child missing in the news, my students will try to locate the girl or boy. They will get bits and pieces of information, like a shallow grave or a tree next to a hill. Maybe they will see the name of a town, but not the state. They might get an image of a child still alive and frightened, or they may get an image of murder. My students become so anxious to tell the police what they've seen, and I understand their enthusiasm because I've felt it myself many times, but—and this is a big but:

Unless you have concrete information, such as the name of the city and the state, the name of the hill, the name of the street where the house is located, the precise place where the body is buried, and so on, the information would not be of interest to the police.

Once upon a time, I kept getting the same dreams of a lost child near where I live in Minnesota, and the policeman I called said he really tried to help me out—and I think he was serious—but he didn't have the manpower to pursue every hunch or vision psychic gets down. He told me that if I really thought I knew where this kid was, I was supposed to go and look for him myself and then call if I found a concrete thing. Despite the immense attention that missing individual cases will generate, it is a sad fact that the police are not always prepared to handle all the data they collect.

The other thing you'll run into is that many police officers believe psychics are frauds. Not everybody believes so; however, many do. Overall, the police would not accept your psychic impressions with open arms. If you turn up unknown at the precinct, they'll be very suspicious—and they should be. They have no excuse not to believe that you are not some "whacko" taking advantage of the situation just to get publicity before you show otherwise. If you want them to take you seriously, you have to give them verifiable, hard proof, some sort of proof that you know what you're talking about.

I'm not going to burst anybody's bubble who feels called to do this kind of job, but you need to know the truth of how it can go. I also met with police forces representatives who were very pleasant and tried to deal with the sketchy bits of information that I gave them. However, even though police welcome your involvement, it's very difficult to get the kind of information needed to locate the boy.

The job itself is very complicated, and I do it only when a member of the family asks me to. Detaching the emotions and pushing away all the information we are fed from the media is not easy. Psychics also automatically get the impression that the person is dead because that's what we see too often in the news.

A few years ago, I recalled a dear friend calling in a panic because her granddaughter was missing for a day. My psychic sense was that the girl was with her boyfriend, who was someone her parents didn't know much about, but my intellect was grappling with that knowledge because another local teen had gone missing about a week ago and had been found murdered. I was hoping that the reality of the situation would be revealed to me, but I did not trust the photos or thoughts that were coming in. The young girl was with her new boyfriend, as it turned out, and she was perfect.

If you are being asked to locate a missing person, my best suggestion is to get just the missing person's name and age. Then leave yourself in a space, ask the Universe to clear you of all preconceived ideas and fears—a high order itself—and then ask the Universe to provide you with clear, specific details that will help you find that individual. If you get a photo of a hill, ask if it is surrounded by something that will help you find it. If you get a town's name, ask for the state. Ask questions about your photos. Now you have to become the detective every inch, to get as many details as you can, but—and that's another major thing:

Only go for the data if anyone asks you to or if you meet someone who can take you seriously in law enforcement. Otherwise, with a lot of potentially useful knowledge and nowhere to go with it, you'll be sitting.

CHAPTER 34:

SOME FINAL TIPS

If you're new to psychic phenomena and you're just learning your own skills, I want to warn you about something that I think is pretty normal, and that goes from one extreme to the next. I went through it with my mom, and I saw some of my students go through it. At the beginning of my and my mother's creation, I recall, we thought that any light that flickered or odd noise that the house-made was some form of spirit world contact. We bought an Ouija board, thinking our psychic creation would be easy. We read everything we could learn about "the supernatural," which is what was named back in the 60s! We went from one end of the pendulum to the other, from having no interest at all in all of this, to immerse ourselves completely in it. This can lead you to burn out easily, however, and in a few instances, I've seen disappointed students try to shut the door entirely on their skills. My recommendation is to take things slowly and to get into all this in moderation. Keep living your life the way you were before you got into psychic growth. In your life, maintain a balance so that you do not burn out. Ultimately, going on a spiritual path and cultivating your spiritual gifts is about cultivating your psychic abilities. It is about a way of thinking and knowing, and here on Earth, you must try to remain grounded in your physical life.

PROVING YOURSELF

The once-famous magician James Randi has made his living as a professional skeptic for as long as I can remember and has put his resources into trying to prove that all psychics are a fraud. He's always questioning psychics, and he claims to keep a check in his pocket for a huge sum of money he'll sign on to the first psychic who can pass a series of tests. I'm not sure what his tests are, but his point is clear: he doesn't think he's ever going to have to cash the check because there are no true psychics.

That guy knows what he's doing. He's a threat to egos, and for everyone, that's a no-win scenario. No doubt, psychics take on his challenge badly, wanting to show him something or two; they want to prove that while humiliating Randi, they are real, and they probably wouldn't mind the cash. However, the whole thing is a setup, and this is what the magician knows. If psychics concentrate on winning a competitive ego contest, they will be blocking themselves from being able to fully use their gifts. Most psychics know better than getting into competitions with skeptics like Randi to "prove it to me." It's inherently a no-win situation, in part, but skeptics are still very proud of being skeptical, and there's nothing that a psychic can do to persuade them of their validity.

If you ever find yourself saying, "I'll show so and so I can do this," or "Just wait and see how good I am," be careful. This means that your ego is in the driver's seat, and most likely, your talents will "fail" you when you think you most need them. There's a lot of James Randis in the world, and our egos are always eager to rise to our defense, but you need to remind yourself that there's nothing you need to prove to anyone. Anyway, skeptics can just see what they want to see. If that sort of circumstance can be avoided, do.

WE'RE NOT FORTUNE COOKIES

Another pit you may often fall into is just showing individuals the data they want to hear. Any people will come to you and want affirmation or reassurance that everything is all right, and you need to be careful not to be swayed by that. Don't turn into one of these psychics who just gives what they want to people. We aren't cookies for fortune.

We're not supposed to vomit out people's happy predictions to make them feel better.

Recently, I received a phone call from a friend whose boyfriend had just broken up with her, and she wanted me to tell her they were going to get back together, and when. Will he call her, and how quickly? Now, what was he thinking? Was he missing her? Has he regretted splitting up?

The timing of her call was so great that I had almost begun to laugh: I was in the middle of writing this advice not to give people what they really wanted to make them feel better. In my third eye came a picture of a stormy path ahead, and I quickly shut it down. I didn't want more details about the woman's issue because she didn't ask for the facts; she wanted me to make her feel better.

"The way they ask their questions, people can try to manipulate the data you send them:" I applied for this job, and I really want it. Can you see it getting me? "The guy I met the other night, and I really want him to call me." Will he and when? "The other day, I felt a lump under my arm, but I'm sure it's nothing. You don't think this is severe, do you? "I have just spent my life savings on a stock that my cousin says is a sure thing." Watch me make a fortune? "I've been trying for four years to get pregnant, and there's nothing going on." I want to have a baby for real. How are you going to see me pregnant?

We don't only get optimistic, happy, cheerful information when we use our gifts to get information about other people's lives. We're opening it up to everyone. Students would often say they just want to carry good knowledge into it, but as psychics, we are not allowed to filter the information we send. When I fell into a bad habit of doing this once, I was alerted by an old psychic friend that knowledge doesn't come to my advantage. It's for the person I'm reading, and I have a responsibility to send whatever data I get to the person. It's not mine to determine what can and can not be done by the person.

The transmission of "bad" details can be very tough. An expectant mother may be asking for her unborn baby, and you may find that the baby has some sort of handicap or does not have a full-term handicap. A client might ask if his spouse cheats on him, hoping you'll say no, but you might see, indeed, the spouse cheats. You could also get the name of the guy with whom his wife has an affair, and that might turn out to be the best friend of the couple. A client could ask about her company, saying she's having some issues, and she wants to know when things are going to turn around. You could get a photo of the individual filing for bankruptcy and losing it all. Another client can inquire about a lump that she can feel in her breast, and you can see it is cancer. Eventually, I found a way out of situations where a customer is too optimistic or even relying on positive responses. When a client asks a very serious question like the above, I ask the person if he or she is open to receiving any details that I receive. I put it back on the customer. If the person says yes, he or she is open to hearing something I have to say, then I continue with the reading and offer what I get to the person.

You would assume that if a client asks a question like the ones mentioned above, then he or she would want to know the truth of the situation, but that's not always the case, I have found. The client would sometimes say, "No, I don't want to hear what you have to say." I just want you to reassure me that my spouse doesn't have an affair, or that my company doesn't go bankrupt, or that I don't have cancer. "Often, when I tell a client that I may not get the details he or she hopes for, the client withdraws that question.

Another thing I found was that if a client tells me to go ahead and send whatever information I receive, and it turns out that the information is "bad," the client generally knows it at a subconscious level and is not shocked at that. If I get details that might be troubling, before saying something, I always double-check it with my guides. Did I correctly perceive it?

Is there something that I really miss? I'm still very cautious because there's nothing I want to misunderstand and therefore offer false hope or false fear. Note, if a person asks a question that could have a difficult answer, ask the person if he or she is open to hearing everything that comes. You'll be shocked by how many people only want to hear positive things in order to make them feel better. It may be human nature, but this is not the role of a psychic.

AVOIDING DEPENDENCY

You also need to look out for individuals who rely on your skills. Some people have no knowledge of their instincts, and from outside of themselves, they are actively seeking guidance and answers. You have to set a cap on how much you think someone can get a reading from you and stick to it (unless something else is said by your intuition). Most of my clients will call me one or two times a year; I'll only get someone who wants to read more than once in a while. When a client becomes reliant on the readings to live his or her life, I can sense, and I instinctively discourage that.

I think this is part of what the Bible speaks about as it warns against "fortune tellers." In order to direct them, people should not rely on psychics, they should trust God, and I agree with that. I agree that there is a fine line between helping and "enabling" people, that is, helping them from taking responsibility for themselves. It is not healthy for either of you to allow others to become dependent on you. Suppose you run into this issue, not if, then, urge people to listen to their own voice inside. There are a variety of books, including my own, A Still Small Voice, on the market that can help people learn how to get in touch with their intuition. As psychics, our task is to help people better understand their lives, not to make ourselves the subject of an individual's life.

FRIENDS AND ACQUANTANCES

You'll probably be practicing on willing friends at the start of your creation, and it'll be fun. Much sharing and several laughs.

Then a common issue is slowly creeping in: your friends could start searching for help with everything in their lives over time. Whenever something comes up that causes them some form of anxiety, fear, or pain, they're going to want you to tell them the result. Your partnerships won't get the same give and take anymore. You may start feeling it's all giving, giving, giving on your part, and you may find yourself totally avoiding your friends.

The other thing that could occur is going to social events. If the word has gotten out that you've improved your psychic abilities, people will come up to you at parties and ask if they can "only ask one psychic question." At first, this may seem interesting, but it gets old, really fast. My recommendation is to immediately nip that in the bud. Let your mates know that you're there to have a nice time like anyone else when you're out socializing with them. Tell them to contact you with their questions at a more suitable time. Another advice is to make some business cards. Then when people ask you for some free psychological advice, give them your business card and tell them to call for a rendezvous. That sounds cold and off-putting, I know, but that's the kind of thing that makes us burn out. Everyone in the world is having some sort of problem, and everyone wants to know how it will work out. If you let anyone you meet become the psychic ATM machine, you'll come to hate them and your gifts.

You have to determine what to do and then set limits and stick to them. There will be moments when your intuition really drives you to send a message to others, and you'll get a definite feeling to stay out of it again. In these instances, follow your instincts and not your intelligence. In the long run, however, just remember that you are still preserving your friendships by shielding yourself.

LET YOUR LIGHT SHINE

In addition to psychic growth and plenty of practice, do you know what the difference is between a "fortune teller" and a "prophet"? It understands that we are deserving of being able to build ourselves to our full potential. It is to discover the strength inside ourselves and to let our light shine.

The more we move into our "Christ-consciousness shoes," the more we recognize and explore our infinite capacity in our oneness with God. We're ceasing to let our fears rule our lives. In order to fit the same mold as everyone else, we quit trying to shrink ourselves. We stop playing small and take on the burden that comes with being God's heir.

The great role models that we have today—John Edward, James Van Praagh, Sylvia Browne, George Anderson, Rosemary Altea—all forced themselves and went up against the lions, so we could see what's possible. I am so grateful to these talented psychics and mediums for growing to the degree they possess and showing us what's possible.

There have been psychically talented people there since the dawn of time. Psychics and mental skills don't go down. Despite what some religions teach, these are Spirit Gifts and should be accepted as such. The Energizer Bunny is the image that pops into my third eye when I think of those presents. Despite all the challenges, we're only moving ahead.

CONCLUSION
Part Two

Thank you for making it through to the end of this book the definitive guide to psychic growth to improve skills such as intuition, clairvoyance, telepathy, healing, reading mediumship, radiating positivity, empath secrets, and communicating to your spirit guides! It should have been insightful, and it should have included all the tools you need to achieve your goals—whatever they might be. The next move is to start using the tips, tricks, tools, and techniques given in this book to start understanding your psychic abilities and become optimistic and motivated as your journey into the psychic power world progresses. You will have the urge to try some of the more challenging strategies and psychic reading styles suggested and mentioned in this book, such as telepathy, crystal ball scrying, mediumship, and aura reading, as you become more confident in your skills and begin to see more results. And remember, practice really makes perfect! But if anything doesn't work right away for you, it doesn't mean it won't work, or you can't use that technique! All can use all of the instruments listed in this book, although it is simpler for others. If you see someone like you who has begun as a beginner but is now better at using a certain practice, it could just come to them more naturally. Don't judge yourself and success on the basis of others—just stick to it, and you'll see how much you're making progress. Moreover, things are likely to come to you more easily than to others, so don't worry—it evens out!

I wish you all the best on your journey and do not forget to learn, to train, and to learn!

Finally, if you find this book helpful in some way, we always appreciate a review on Amazon!

Made in the USA
Middletown, DE
25 April 2021